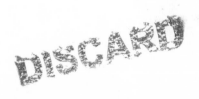

Health Maintenance Through Physical Conditioning

Edited by Robert C. Cantu, MD

PSG Publishing Company, Inc. • *Littleton, Massachusetts*

Library of Congress Cataloging in Publication Data

Main entry under title:

Health maintenance through physical conditioning.

  Bibliography: p.
  Includes index.
  1. Sports medicine. 2. Health. 3. Physical
fitness. 4. Sports--Accidents and injuries--
Prevention. I. Cantu, Robert C. [DNLM:
1. Health promotion. 2. Physical fitness.
3. Sports medicine. QT255 H4334]
RC1210.H38   613.7'1   80-15622
ISBN 0-88416-312-1

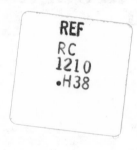
Printed in the United States of America.

International Standard Book Number: 0-88416-312-1

Library of Congress Catalog Card Number: 80-15622

CONTRIBUTORS

Robert Burns Arnot, MD, CM
Consultant Physician, Sports Physiology
Eighteenth Olympic Winter Games
Lake Placid, New York

Robert C. Cantu, MA, MD, FACS
Chief, Neurosurgical Service and
Chairman, Department of Surgery
Emerson Hospital
Concord, Massachusetts

Henry D. Childs, MD
Department of Medicine
Emerson Hospital
Concord, Massachusetts

Earl F. Hoerner, MD, MPH
Director, Sportsmedicine and Ambulatory Care
Braintree Hospital
Braintree, Massachusetts

Lyle J. Micheli, MD
Director, Division of Sports Medicine
Children's Hospital Medical Center
Boston, Massachusetts

Harriet G. Tolpin, PhD
Associate Professor of Economics
Simmons College
Boston, Massachusetts

Paul Vinger, MD
Harvard Medical School
Boston, Massachusetts and
Emerson Hospital
Concord, Massachusetts

Medicine is an ever-changing science. As new research and clinical experience broaden our knowledge, changes in treatment and drug therapy are required. The editor and the publisher of this work have made every effort to ensure that the treatment and drug dosage schedules herein are accurate and in accord with the standards accepted at the time of publication. Readers are advised, however, to check the product information sheet included in the package of each drug they plan to administer to be certain that changes have not been made in the recommended dose or in the indications and contraindications for administration. This recommendation is of particular importance in regard to new or infrequently used drugs.

CONTENTS

ACKNOWLEDGEMENTS

I would like to express my special thanks to Bernice McPhee, Director of Education and Training at Emerson Hospital, her Administrative Assistant Elaine Leone, and staff Pauline McCabe, Instructor, and Gretchen Ellis, Assistant Instructor. Their superb help made possible this seminar and resultant publication. I would also like to acknowledge the men of the Keith Vocational High School who videotaped the seminar, and finally Pat Blackey, my secretary, whose skills so facilitated the preparation of this manuscript.

INTRODUCTION

The decade of the 1970s will be remembered for many things, good and bad. A war most of our country emotionally could not support in Vietnam, the resignation of President Nixon to escape criminal prosecution, and gas lines as petroleum prices tripled in less than two years stand out on the negative side. On the positive side was an affirmation of equal opportunity for all as exemplified by the continuing civil rights and women's liberation movements.

As a physician, perhaps the most exciting positive development was the realization that just as Niccolo Machiavelli had said in *The Prince* in 1513, "fortune is the arbiter of half the things we do, leaving the other half or so to be controlled by ourselves." This concept was dramatically illustrated by the concern for physical fitness and the concept of "preventive medicine," or what I choose to call health maintenance. The message was read loud and clear that our three major killers of the seventies, heart disease, cancer, and diabetes, all are largely the result of an inappropriate life-style (inactivity and obesity), and self-pollution (smoking, alcohol, and drug abuse).

The response was dramatic as millions of Americans engaged in a fitness mania as the tennis boom gave way to a tidal wave of running. While basically positive, this overenthusiastic, under-informed, excessive headlong dash into fitness has many potential hazards. Just as deaths were attributed to various dietary extreme "fad diets," so, too, a similar end befell others too vigorously pursuing exercise. Thus, sports medicine services sprang up at hospitals to treat the flood of overuse musculo-skeletal injuries seen primarily in adult "recreational athletes."

As fitness has become a popular topic, quite naturally the media have given it considerable coverage. Unfortunately, the more sensational aspects (the winner plus a shot of the fifteen thousand in the New York Marathon), half-truths, and just plain myths have been propagated by the media. Athletes, laypersons, paramedical, and even some medical personnel, all without a proper exercise physiology background, are expounding on topics where they lack expertise.

Today, as the 1980s begin, those in sports medicine must accept the challenge to educate the nation's coaches, trainers, physical therapists, and competitive and recreational athletes in applying "pure" knowledge to the "practical" problems of improving performance while avoiding injury. Notable among the new subdivisions in sports medicine providing such information are sports physiology, psychology, nutrition, and biomechanics. Furthermore, we must accept the responsibility of providing safe exercise programs for health maintenance for society as a whole. The only practical way to reduce health care spending is to decrease dollars spent on its major drain—hospitalization. Since our leading causes of death and disability are largely preventable through changes in life-style, nutrition, and self-pollution, the goal is clearly attainable.

This effort is directed at giving such essential information to you, athletes, trainers, coaches, medical personnel, and laypersons. Each section is contributed by a doctor with practical expertise in that area. Each of us has a burning conviction to present only the unblemished facts, while exposing the many myths. I trust at the conclusion that you will feel our goal has been attained.

1 Physical Conditioning of the Cardiovascular System and the Scientific Basis of the Marathon and Other Endurance Sports

Robert Burns Arnot, MD

Our first author has a bibliography that reads like a Who's Who of exercise physiology laboratories throughout the world. Equally at home at an academic meeting, in a radio or TV studio, or piloting his twin-engine plane above snowcapped mountains, he is currently the Director of the Exercise Physiology Laboratories at Lake Placid and Consultant Physiologist to our 1980 Winter Olympics Team. His initial presentation is on the physical conditioning of the cardiovascular system and scientific basis of the marathon.

With a population of 17 million people East Germany won 47 gold medals in the 1976 Olympic Games, the United States only 40. Much of their success is due to a national sports medicine program. Beginning in Leipzig during the early fifties, a sports and sports science institute was founded as an outgrowth of "scientific socialism" aimed at population fitness. In 1965 the focus shifted to Olympic sport, putting East Germany on the map in 1968 at Mexico City. By 1976 in Montreal, 17 sports centers had been established, with 1000 to 2000 athletes at each, containing sports sciences appropriate to specialty events. A strong grass roots program of education and testing was established through a comprehensive club program.

Athletes are often identified by parents or teachers through a bonus system. To harvest the "natural athlete" from such a small population, certain sports developed screening techniques. As early as age 3 gymnasts' potentials are examined through special motor skills testing. An electromyogram (EMG) muster pattern is specific for sprinters at age 5. Anthropometric data of webbing in hands and feet are characteristic for swimmers by 6.

Athletes have a very specific individualized training program that includes prevention of over-training syndromes and the injuries that have plagued US athletes. As we observe the East German athlete starting at the age of 3 or 4 through their athletic career we have a vivid example of what happens to an individual's cardiovascular system as extreme fitness is achieved.

The Heart

We begin, of course, with the heart. Today we realize that the observed training changes have less to do with the heart than initially thought. The cardiac changes that occur in a 12- or 13-year-old child beginning an endurance program, such as long-distance running, are different from those who enter a pressure sport, like wrestling or weight lifting. These changes require about eight years of training. Twelve- and thirteen-year-old children are about age 20 or 21 before they have full development of their cardiac systems.

The training effects that we see remain controversial. Some exercise physiologists contend the heart increases in contractility, and it is certainly true that when a trained heart is in a hypoxic situation under a tremendous pressure load it is able to maintain a greater contractility than an untrained heart. The biggest changes in the heart are seen in the volume of the main pumping chamber, the left ventricle. Marathon runners, or athletes involved in an endurance sport, will experience large increases in the volume of the left ventricle. The left ventricular mass also increases, but compared to the pressure sport athlete, the ventricular wall is thinner and the chamber larger.

Controversy remains about whether or not the coronary arteries enlarge in response to endurance training. Since a lot of athletes have not been autopsied we are really not certain. It is interesting to note though that Clarence DeMar, Mr Boston Marathon, who won that event seven times and who met an untimely death at age 66 from cancer of the stomach, had very large coronary arteries at autopsy. Interestingly he had considerable coronary artery atherosclerotic disease. Thus the unequivocal training effects on the heart are three: an increase in end diastolic volume, increased left ventricular mass, and perhaps an increase in contractility. The increase in left ventricular mass is greatest for the pressure athlete. Imagine a wrestler trying to hold an individual for 30 or 40 seconds or a weight lifter trying to lift 300 or 400 lb; the heart has an obligation to maintain a tremendous pressure head, and the effect is the development of a very thick left ventricular wall without an increase in chamber size.

On x-ray the pressure athlete's heart is no larger than the sedentary nonathlete's. Many years ago, essentially with the development of the x-ray, endurance athletes were noted to have hearts larger than the population at large. In the 1930s scientists in Shanghai noticed that rickshaw drivers had large hearts. The businessmen who were being carried around had normal-sized hearts. They thought they were being saved from this disastrous athlete's heart. Well, they found out 40 years later that this was not the case as the rickshaw drivers long outlived the businessmen they pulled around. Numerous Swiss studies of teenagers confirm that during this age period it requires about eight years for maximal cardiac conditioning. For those of us adults who begin training later in life, the same cardiac changes occur but take place over a shorter period of time, about two or three years.

Conductance

Perhaps the greatest recent advances have been in learning what happens to the cardiac output after it leaves the heart. There are two very dramatic findings. The first regards vascular conductance. The sedentary individual has a very high peripheral resistance as he begins to exercise. The well-conditioned athlete, quite the opposite, has a very low peripheral resistance or a very high conductance. An example is the runner or cross-country skier who has well-trained lower extremities. The sympathetic control of the peripheral vasculature has really released a certain amount of tone so that there is an increase in conductance. There is also an increase in capillarization (Figure 1-1), the number of smaller blood vessels. The main effect of endurance training is a decrease in sympathetic tone and resultant increase in conductance. Thus there is a low peripheral resistance and a relatively low work load on the heart in terms of the pressure against which it has to pump. A runner who does no upper body work will have high conductance in the legs only. This same individual when shoveling snow with untrained upper extremities will experience a tremendous increase in pressure. That is why coronary care units often fill up after a snowstorm with individuals who might walk or perhaps even jog. They have subjected their hearts to pressure loads far surpassing accustomed levels.

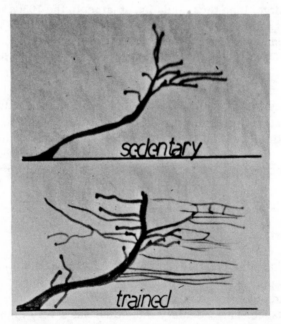

Figure 1-1 Drawing of increased capillarization that occurs in a trained individual.

Recently we have observed an interesting new finding in our Olympic-caliber cross-country skiers. Their lower extremities are well trained with a very low peripheral resistance–very high conductance to blood flow from the heart. However, when we look at their upper extremities we find relatively low conductance and high total peripheral resistance. Thus we observe they actually lose power when they start to use their arms in addition to legs, as when going up a hill. Last spring when we tested our Olympic cross-country ski team at my laboratory, I found that only Bill Koch and Alison Ellen Spencer, our best female skier, were able to, in effect, add arms and legs together without a loss of power.

Maximum Oxygen Consumption

Maximum oxygen consumption is the measurement of one's greatest capacity to consume oxygen. For any of you who have been in or read about endurance athletics you must realize that this, the VO_2 max, is a number the athletes seem to focus on. Crew and cross-country ski team members, when asked what kind of shape they are in, will answer they are a 74 or 76. In Scandinavia that number is known as the condition's number, and if someone asked you what kind of shape you were in and you replied 80, they would know you were in tremendous shape. The highest score ever recorded was 94 by Sveno-Oke Lundbeck, the great Swedish cross-country ski racer. United States national cross-country team members are in the low 80s. Marathon runner Bill Rogers is 78 and Frank Shorter 70. The population at large is in the 40s and Alpine ski racers in the 50s.

To determine maximum oxygen consumption—the best overall assessment of cardiovascular fitness—we must find how effectively muscle is able to extract oxygen from the blood going by. The sum total of the heart, lungs, blood vessels, and muscle interaction is reflected in the maximum oxygen consumption. In Figure 1-2 Dr Cantu is being tested in my laboratory. The nose is blocked, so he is able to inhale through a top valve and exhale through a bottom valve. The exhaled air is continuously monitored for oxygen and carbon dioxide concentration. Knowing the oxygen concentration being inspired, a computer gives a

5

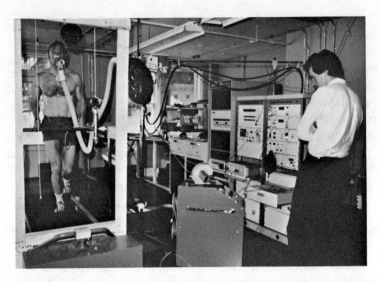

Figure 1-2 Laboratory treadmill ergometer for determining VO$_2$ max.

continuous readout of the oxygen consumed. The heart rate is also monitored and fed through an analog digital converter. The computer has eliminated the need for having 5, 6, or even 7 laboratory technicians to collect exhaled air bags and sample the concentrations of gases in them.

A rowing ergometer, bicycle ergometer, or cross-country ski simulator using the arms and legs together can be used with the same computer setup. This affords the opportunity to assess conductance. An example is a cross-country skier whose oxygen consumption for legs alone is 70 and arms alone is 50. When looked at together they are not simply additive. When this individual exercises with arms and legs together, there is a tremendous increase in total peripheral resistance. We actually find the oxygen consumption is 66 so there is not an increase in oxygen consumption but actually a decrease in power. While this is an indirect method it is nonetheless a very nice way of getting relatively precise information with which to plan training regimens for athletes. The Scandinavians and East Germans have even designed swimming flumes where the water runs through at a known speed and the swimmer's oxygen consumption is calculated.

It is important to realize that you must be testing the specific muscle groups involved. If an athlete were using only his arms, he could have a tremendously large heart, large lungs, and a great total peripheral resistance; yet such a small muscle mass would be involved that he would not have a very high oxygen consumption. There is a wide variety of different mixes of arms, legs, trunk, abdomen, etc that will be used by an elite-class athlete.

Muscle

What has been personally the most fascinating part of this whole field is muscle physiology. So far we have been able to come from the heart, through the conducting system, to the actual site where oxygen is extracted and used. Tremendous advances have occurred during the last decade. We are able to select the kind of sport an individual should probably go into based on muscle type as determined by muscle biopsy. About 15 years ago a method was developed by Bergstrom using a 4 mm needle to obtain a sample of muscle for microscopic examination. The actual procedure involves anesthetizing the skin and subcutaneous layer of fat and fascia overlying the muscle. The skin is nicked with a #11 surgical blade and the 4 mm biopsy needle is inserted into the muscle. I can assure you that this does not hurt. A small piece of muscle is extracted from which considerable information about the athlete can be obtained. Figure 1-3 is an example of such a section of muscle under the microscope.

There are two fiber types, the darker fast-twitch fibers and the lighter gray slow-twitch fibers. A higher proportion of fast-twitch fibers is characteristic of a sprint athlete while the slow-twitch predominate in the endurance athlete. The general sedentary population has approximately 50% slow-twitch, 50% fast-twitch, as does the power-sport athlete—discus, javelin, shotput, weight lifting, etc. The slower twitch fibers are used to control and direct the javelin or shotput and the fast-twitch for the power and the extreme acceleration required.

These patterns are probably present from birth. Studies of identical twins have shown they have identical fiber types. In

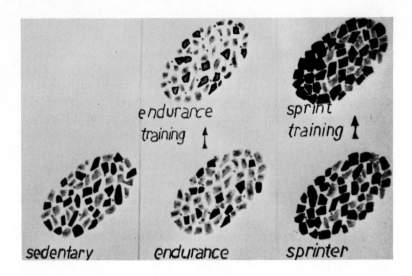

Figure 1-3 Muscle samples from biopsy showing the various combinations of fast-twitch and slow-twitch fibers.

fact, looking at the entire cardiopulmonary system we find almost no difference between monozygous twins except for the muscular system, where developmental differences are seen depending on training. Superior sprinters are born with 70% or even 80% fast-twitch fibers. They have a relatively low capacity to consume oxygen but high capacity to do speed work. Such an individual may be able to run a 100-meter dash but would probably never finish a marathon.

Last year we studied Andy Young, who was a fine high school sprinter. He had approximately 80% fast-twitch fibers and even to this day can run a tremendously fast 100- to 220-meter dash. He is unable, however, to finish even a 10,000-meter fun run. His muscles have very little ability to consume oxygen, but with all these fast-twitch fibers, extreme capacity to do aerobic power (sprint) work. With power training these fast-twitch fibers become even larger and the latest evidence indicates that they will even split so that an increase in fast-twitch fibers and muscle bulk occurs. Individuals with primarily slow-twitch fibers can lift weights with a resultant very modest increase in muscle bulk while one with primarily fast-twitch fibers rapidly takes on a Charles Atlas figure in response to weight lifting. This is because of the ability of the fast-twitch fiber to dramatically increase in size, something the slow-twitch fiber just cannot do.

The superior endurance athlete is born with a high percentage of slow-twitch endurance fibers that have the ability to consume oxygen. If they start training in their early teens a maximal heart size will be achieved by the age of 20 or 21. The specific training effects realized over the ensuing 10 to 20 years occur almost entirely in the muscle. The endurance fibers of the elite endurance athlete may actually become a little smaller, decreasing the distance oxygen has to travel to get to that cell. There is also a dramatic increase in the number of capillaries so the blood flow to the muscle is enhanced. It is not certain whether this is an increase in capillaries or whether they actually double back on each other. This greatly enhances the capacity of the muscle to extract oxygen. More capillaries, smaller muscle cells, and an increase in the number of mitochondrial enzymes to extract that oxygen are the major changes in response to years of endurance training.

We have mentioned the natural selection in terms of the fiber type that one is born with; yet some changes do occur in fast-twitch fibers in response to volume training. They do not turn into slow-twitch fibers but do increase their ability to consume oxygen and thus accomplish an endurance event. This happens with distance or tempo training. Thus, actually four changes occur in the muscle as a result of volume training: an increase in capillaries, decrease in slow-twitch fiber size, increase in mitochondria, and a change in the fast-twitch fibers with an increase in their ability to consume oxygen.

Recently further advances have come with the use of the electron microscope and analysis of individual muscle enzymes. A single muscle fiber is cut into over 15 different pieces and each enzyme and its biochemical pathway, be it glycolytic or Krebs cycle itself, is identified. The slow-twitch fiber or endurance fiber has many mitochondria. As this individual has trained, the cell has become slightly smaller and the mitochondrion increases dramatically in size. In contrast the fast-twitch fibers have few mitochondria and thus a very low ability to consume oxygen. They may have large glycogen stores that they can rapidly utilize, but at the expense of a buildup of lactic acid that brings the ability of the muscle to contract to a halt. The mitochondria thus limit the ability of the muscle cell to work aerobically, and their increase in response to endurance training is of paramount importance.

The store of glycogen in the cell is studied to counsel the endurance athlete on the optimal training program. After an individual's tempo training run in which he has gone 40 or 45 minutes at race pace, the muscle is virtually depleted of glycogen. The next day's training should be at a more leisurely pace. As it turns out even in the world's best athletes it takes about 48 hours, and for most of us a minimum of 72 hours, before the muscle glycogen is restored. For some it may be five or six days. By studying the glycogen content it can thus be determined how long it takes the individual athlete to restore the glycogen and thus determine how frequently to pursue hard training runs. For most this will be every third day.

Thus far in response to endurance training we have discussed the adaptation of the heart (enlargement), lungs (better oxygen uptake), and muscle (smaller slow-twitch fibers, increase in fast-twitch fibers' ability to consume oxygen, and increase in mitochondria).

The Brain and the Anaerobic Threshold

The brain's adaptation as reflected by an increase in anaerobic threshold is one of the most important responses to volume training after age 20. A very brief run through of what the anaerobic threshold looks like starts with the brain. From the motor cortex a stimulus comes down through the spinal cord, out through an individual nerve to the neuromuscular junction where the impulse actually reaches the muscle cell, and tells it to perform its work. The anaerobic threshold is determined by the buildup of lactic acid. Those of you who exercise recognize this as the tightness, the burning in muscle, and the shortness of breath that comes at a specific point in your exertion. If it is a 100-meter dash, it is probably the last 10 meters or so. If it is a marathon, it might be the top of a hill where you are pushing a little bit too hard.

What is happening is that work demands exceed the capacity for muscle to aerobically function through glycolysis in the Krebs cycle. Thus, instead, anaerobic pathways are used with a buildup of lactic acid (Figure 1-4). There are two instances where

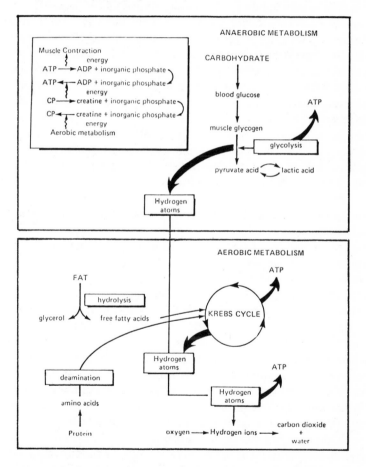

Figure 1-4 Simplified schematic drawing of anaerobic and aerobic metabolism, with ATP energy formation, in a single muscle cell.

lactic acidosis rises rapidly. The first is at the onset of exercise when the delivery of increased oxygen has not had a chance to occur. The gun goes off starting a 100-meter dash or someone runs up behind you on a dark street requiring your speedy exit. The body has not had a chance to respond and would be able to break down glycogen only to the point of pyruvic acid, and with inadequate oxygen around, lactic acid is formed. The second case and perhaps the most interesting, which tells us about training effects, has to do with the actual threshold for lactic acidosis.

Those who studied traditional physiology will remember teachers talking about aerobic and anaerobic work. Aerobic really has to do with the ability of oxygen to be extracted by muscle and to do useful work by the Krebs cycle. Anaerobic occurs when there is not enough oxygen around. In the first case when the individual is being attacked or trying to run a 100-meter dash that is true. But it is not true when an individual tries to increase his pace. Walking across a room an athlete may recruit or activate perhaps only 20% of his muscle fibers. As he progresses from a walk to a fast jog more muscle fibers are recruited. At this pace only aerobic slow-twitch fibers are activated so all the work is done by the Krebs cycle. Finally at a sprint pace the fast-twitch anaerobic fibers are recruited and a dramatic increase in lactic acid results.

There are specific training measures to increase the point at which lactic acidosis occurs. We find that if athletes train at or below the anaerobic threshold that muscular injuries and minor ills that impede performance are avoided. We also find that by aerobic tempo training the athlete can increase the amount of work accomplished before the anaerobic threshold is reached. World-class athletes as they come to the finish line or push over the top of a hill have a pH inside their cells of about 6.5 while the lowest seen in untrained individuals is about 6.9. With this tremendous increase in acidity (lactic acidosis) cells actually stop functioning and one grinds to a halt, the phenomenon we see at the top of Heartbreak Hill in the Boston Marathon.

Training well below the anaerobic threshold there is little improvement in performance. Those who train for marathons with only long, slow distance find no increase in speed unless they also run some short races. On the other hand, the individual doing a lot of interval training at short tempo, that is 5 or 10 minutes at all-out race pace, probably is injured much more but gains in speed. The philosophy of the Harvard Track Team in previous years has been to run the athletes as hard and as long as they can and whoever survives goes to the meet. By being able to train at or around the anaerobic threshold a very dramatic increase in this threshold occurs month by month. This is much more important, obviously, for the elite-class, high school, or college athletes than it is for patients being tested or individuals being counseled in a fitness program. But it does have several applications: first, you really do not want to exceed the anaerobic threshold, second, you do not want to push near that level more than one day out of three.

There are a very few key indicators of one's state of fitness. The first is the VO_2 max—the maximum oxygen consumption. This affords one idea of what an athlete's potential is, ie, what he has been able to develop over his childhood years, or, for the middle-aged athlete, the first three years of an endurance training program. The second indicator of conditioning is the anaerobic threshold or how much of that oxygen consumption can be used.

To emphasize this Frank Shorter, one of America's best marathon runners until his injury, will be used as an example. Frank won the Olympic gold medal in 1972 and the silver medal in 1976, yet he has a relatively low oxygen consumption. Remember the top number we spoke about was 94; many cross-country ski racers are in the 80s; Bill Rogers is a 78; but Frank Shorter's VO_2 max is only 70. However, he is able to use fully 90% of that oxygen before reaching his anaerobic threshold, a tremendously high level. Bill Rogers uses only about 80% or 82% of his oxygen consumption before reaching his anaerobic threshold. For the untrained athlete only 60% of the oxygen consumption can be utilized before lactic acidosis ensues. A third indicator of conditioning is the speed with which the system can deliver oxygen, how rapidly an individual can take oxygen from the air and deliver it to the muscle cell. For most this takes 2 to 3 minutes to occur.

For the population at large a less sophisticated measurement of training is the oxygen pulse—the heart rate at which a specific amount of oxygen is consumed. With endurance training an athlete will attain a lower and lower heart rate at the same oxygen consumption level. This is because of several different factors. In the past most thought it was due to the heart alone. The heart increases in cardiac output, stroke volume, and contractility, but this is a small part of the whole picture. The total peripheral resistance decreases, and conductance increases, allowing more blood to be pumped from the heart. Also there is an increase in oxygen extraction.

In conclusion, it is important to realize how quickly these effects of endurance training are lost by inactivity. I think it is important for athletes and individuals supervising sports programs (especially for patients rehabilitating from an illness) to realize that within 2 to 3 weeks of inactivity one loses about 20% of conditioning and in about a month as much as 50%. Thus it is lost much, much more quickly than it is gained and it takes an even longer period to get it back again. Thus the message is clear for athletes and those of us exercising for our health as well; training is a year-round proposition, with ideally no hiatus of more than a few days.

SUGGESTED READINGS

Bruce, R., and DeRouen, T. Exercise testing as a predictor of heart disease and sudden death. *Hosp Pract.* 13:69–75, 1978.

Cohn, K., Kamm, B., Feteih, N., et al. The use of treadmill score to quantify ischemic response and to predict extent of coronary disease. *Circulation* 59:386–296, 1979.

Engel, G.L. Psychologic stress, vasodepressor (Vasovag) syncope, and sudden death. *Ann Intern Med.* 89:403–412, 1978.

Epstein, S. Value and limitations of the electrocardiographic response to exercise in assessment of patients with coronary artery disease. *Am J Cardiol.* 48:667–673, 1978.

Froelicher, B.F., Thompson, A.J., Longo, M.R., et al. Value of exercise testing for screening asymptomatic men for latent coronary disease. *Prog Cardiovasc Dis.* 18:265–276, 1976.

Kramer, N., Susamano, A., and Shekelle, R.B. The "false-negative" treadmill exercise test and left ventricular dysfunction. *Circulation* 57:763–768, 1978.

Levites, R., and Anderson, G. Detection of critical coronary lesions with treadmill exercise testing: fact or fiction? *Am J Cardiol.* 42:533–538, 1978.

Morris, S., and McHenry, P. Role of exercise stress testing in healthy subjects and patients with coronary heart disease. *Am J Cardiol.* 42:659–666, 1978.

Lozener, B., and Morganroth, J. New criteria to enhance the predictability of coronary artery disease by exercise testing in asymptomatic subjects. *Circulation* 56:799–802, 1977.

Selzer, A., Cohn, K., and Goldschlager, N. On the interpretation of exercise test. *Circulation* 58:103–105, 1978.

Siegel, W., Blomquist, G., and Mitchell, J.H. Effects of a quantified physical training program on middle-aged sedentary men. *Circulation* 41:19–29, 1970.

2 Exercise and Life-style Modification in Family Practice

Henry D. Childs, MD

The next chapter was written by a fellow Emerson Hospital physician who is one of the pioneers in what one day, I hope, will be commonplace in medical practice. Dr Childs perhaps exemplifies best what all of us today believe in and are trying to accomplish: give you the knowledge to live healthier, happier, more productive, injury-free lives. He has devoted a major portion of his family practice time counseling patients how to avoid illness, rather than just treating those already afflicted. Now you become the patient as you listen to Dr Henry Childs discuss Exercise and Life-style Modification in Family Practice.

I find that in trying to train and condition people, changing life-style is the name of the game. People must first realize that there are problems and the physician must make them understand that there are active changes that need to be accomplished. I do not like to emphasize negatives, but we must start off with the fact that in our society at large we have these problems.

Think of it perhaps as rusting-degenerative diseases, problems that, to a greater or lesser degree, affect all of us (Table 2-1). Obesity—look around any public gathering; how many people are at least a little paunchy, a little overweight, show evidence of deconditioning? Generalized atherosclerosis is a major problem in our society; coronary artery disease, an offshoot of that, is our biggest killer. Essential hypertension is a major problem. It is a crippler as many strokes develop from hypertension and are thus preventable. Maturity-onset (noninsulin-dependent) diabetes is slowly coming out of hiding, and although not entirely preventable, it is a common problem.

Table 2-1
The Human Junkyard
Rusting-degenerative diseases and/or other affiliated problems that are contributed to by poor life-style

---

Obesity
Generalized atherosclerosis
Coronary artery disease
Essential hypertension
Maturity-onset (noninsulin-dependent) diabetes
Hyperlipidemias (especially low HDL, high LDL)
Symptomatic osteoarthritis (other arthritides?)
Osteoporosis
Chronic fatigue and lethargy (accompanied by the "let somebody else do it" syndrome)
Chronic depression and anxiety states
Poor job performance due to mental and physical deconditioned status
Unnecessary injuries or illnesses due to poor overall condition
Stress-related symptoms (over 70% of presenting complaints in patients under 50 in most primary care practices include tension headaches and neckaches, back and chest pain, functional abdominal distress)
Chronic obstructive pulmonary disease (COPD) and other smoking-related diseases
Marital, family, sexual maladjustments—eventual severe reactive depressions, alcoholism, drug dependency, suicide
Postretirement involution (decreased mental, physical, and social activity)

Many of these areas that we are looking at are affected by heredity. But the question we must keep in mind is even if some of these problems are going to ultimately occur, to what degree can they be stalled or made milder?

Hyperlipidemias   Current knowledge suggests problems with not only the hyperlipoproteinemias, but also the concept that the low-high density ratio of cholesterol is important. It appears that the low-density lipoproteins cause an increase in atherosclerosis, and the high-density lipoproteins are protective.

Symptomatic osteoarthritis   This disease certainly is affected by deconditioning and a sedentary life-style. Any rheumatologist will tell you that no matter what the predisposition may be, good, regular sustained physical activity reduces the symptoms and keeps them at bay longer. The same is true for other arthritides as well.

Osteoporosis   This disease, affecting mainly the elderly, is one of the fascinating areas that Dr Arnot has some comments on later. We are beginning to study preventive medicine for the geriatric age groups. There are some very preliminary word-of-mouth reports beginning to come out. As we look at people in their sixties and seventies being fitness-trained to masters'levels of running, cross-country skiing, swimming, and other aerobic activities, we are finding changes in body fat, potassium, carbohydrate, and calcium metabolism, degree of osteoporosis, control of hypertension, and reduced incidence of heart attack, among other areas.

Many are now aware of the study at Harvard by Dr Paffenbarger et al that demonstrates a definite drop-off in the incidence of heart attacks in individuals exercising to a level of 2000 kilocalories per week. Carried out over ten years, it is a highly significant study.[1]

The chronic fatigue and lethargy ("let somebody else do it") syndrome has a great deal of reflection socially. Chronic depression and anxiety states, and poor job performance may be due to deconditioned mental and physical states. Unnecessary injuries or illness may result from poor overall conditioning and stress-related symptoms. In a primary care practice, this can represent over 70% of the problems encountered.

A question any primary care doctor must ponder is whether the patient's symptoms reflect organic disease or rather are stress-related? Second, at this particular point in the individual's life, did this really have to happen? Is it unavoidable, or is it, frankly, a matter of poor life-style, ie, cigarette smoking, marital, family, and sexual maladjustments, reactive depression, suicide, alcoholism, or drug dependency? Postretirement involution is another major problem. Once people are on the shelf at 65 or earlier, the rusting process may not only be physical, but social and mental as well. These are areas that I think are of great concern to all of us.

In talking to my patients, I liken all of this to a swamp into which the average person is slowly sagging down. In the past five years addressing these problems, I often ask my patients at their initial visit, "What percentage of my patients do you think are really in excellent health, meaning no organic disease and are also in excellent physical condition using Kenneth Cooper's 30 aerobic points per week test?" The guesses run anywhere from 10% to 50%. Although I do not keep accurate books on it, it actually has been closer to 0.5% to 1%. So, it is a relatively small percentage of the population, at least as I have come across them in five years, who are operating anywhere near optimum performance.

A number of years ago, when I still understood what was happening under the hood of my car and worked on it, I walked into a large junkyard, looking for a part for my car. In one corner of this junkyard I came across an old Rolls Royce—a Silver Cloud that could have been worth 70 to 80 thousand dollars. It was all rusted out, and had birds' nests inside of it; the handsewn leather interior was gone and the exterior in utter ruin as well. When you see one of the most magnificent machines that mankind has made in this condition, it is really a rather horrifying experience. You have to ask yourself, how could somebody possibly let a machine as nice as this, which had years of elegant life left, go completely to pieces? It really boggles the mind! In the primary care situation, there is an obvious analogy to patients. Although many patients see the direct analogy they do not realize that primary care doctors, in every day of their practices are walking through a junkyard filled with human wreckage! If the Rolls Royce is thought of as a nice machine, you cannot begin to compare it to this one that we have all inherited. The owning and operating of this machine for a number of years, and its proper maintenance, is something that I think should be prized highly.

LIFE-STYLE ANALYSIS

How do you alert the average patient to the problem? This can be done in two ways. I view any contact a patient makes with me as an opportunity to at least lay the groundwork to get started on his or her problem. Naturally, it boils down at first to life-style analysis. This starts at the initial visit. Table 2-2 indicates the things we look at when a patient comes in with a medical problem. Naturally, if somebody is sick and hurting, you cannot spend a great deal of time with generalities, you have to address the problem. At the first visit documentation of age, sex, occupation, smoking history, diet pattern and quality, current or past regular exercise habits and types, known medical or surgical conditions, current or past regular medications (including over-the-counter drugs, which are important also), known allergies, and significant family history is made. This does not take much time to elucidate and can be accomplished by the physician, nurse, or secretary.

Table 2-2
Life-style Analysis

Initial visit (usually for a medical problem)

    Identify: Age, sex, occupation, smoking history, brief diet pattern and quality, any current or past regular exercise habit and type; known medical or surgical conditions; current or past regular medications (including OTCs); known allergies; significant family history

Complete history and physical examination

    Occupational history, job satisfaction

    Present worries, problems, symptoms

    Past medical history (including hospitalizations, operations, significant injuries, past disabilities, allergies, medications, infectious illnesses, immunizations, foreign travel, military service duty and locations, special tests)

    Family medical history

    Social history (type and location of residence, how many moves, marital/sexual satisfaction, concerns about children, family planning, hobbies and other interests and activities outside job, how much sleep, diet quality and pattern in some detail, type and regularity of exercise, smoking history, alcohol pattern and amount, drug use or abuse)

    Review of systems

    Physical examination

    Basic screening blood and urine testing, resting ECG

    Special testing as indicated by age, sex, identified problems (stress ECG, fasting lipid profile, glucose tolerance test)

At the end of the complete physical examination, delineate all significant problems, but also assess state of health (presence or absence of organic or emotional disease) and physical condition by comparison with current standards of regular aerobic exercise (over 2000 kcal/week)

If you really are going to try to convince a person to change his life-style significantly, you can intrigue, interest, and point out problems quickly in this setting. But the ideal vehicle, I think, is the complete history and physical examination, which allows you not only to go over in more detail what the various problems are but to do some teaching.

Briefly, as I see a complete history and physical examination, the basic factors are: an occupational history and job satisfaction report, present worries, symptoms, and problems, and past medical history. The medical history is taken by most physicians and includes: operations, hospitalizations, significant injuries, past disabilities, allergies, medications, infectious illnesses, immunizations, foreign travel, military service duty and locations, and special tests. A family medical history is, of course, important.

Social history is the most important part of the routine or specialized history and physical examination because here are noted: type and location of residence, how many homes, marital and sexual satisfaction, concerns about children, family planning, hobbies, other interests and activities outside of the job, how much sleep, diet quality and pattern in some detail, type and regularity of exercise, smoking history, alcohol pattern and amount, and drug use or abuse. In other words, this is where patients really live, and this is where I spend the most time. A review of systems is taken, of course; finally a physical examination, whatever basic screening blood and urine testing seem indicated, and a resting ECG are taken.

At this point, having gone over the above, special testing may be indicated by the patient's age, sex, or any identified problems. A fasting lipid profile, glucose tolerance test, and a stress ECG may all be pertinent. At the end of this particular examination it is important not only to delineate for your patient all the significant problems that you have uncovered, but also to assess both the state of health (which means simply the presence or absence of organic or emotional disease) and the patient's physical condition. If you have taken a detailed exercise history, it is relatively easy to compare this with the known aerobic standards. In my practice, I use the 2000 kcal per week standard for aerobic exercise. You can tell patients where they stand with regard to a very good standard of preventive medicine and what you assess their physical condition and general health to be. It is thus a dynamic analysis.

Assessing Risk Factors

Assessing risk factors is really part of the foregoing (Table 2-3). A family history of cardiac disease and/or hyperlipidemia is of concern. The young cardiac death syndrome—the man who never knew his father or had a brother die at age 35 or 40, tips one off to the need for a fasting lipoprotein phenotyping with an HDL/LDL cholesterol ratio. Triglyceride levels are meaningful only in the fasting state. Thus the lipoprotein screens should be done after a 12 to 14 hour fast. The most convenient way of doing that is by having the patient eat supper by 7 PM and consume nothing but water during the night, then take the test first thing in the morning.

Table 2-3
Assessing Risk Factors

Family history of cardiac disease and/or hyperlipidemia
Family and/or personal history of heavy smoking, alcohol abuse
Overweight
Poor diet quality and pattern
Sedentary life-style
Hypertension
Prediabetic or established diabetic status
Hyperlipoproteinemia, and/or high triglycerides, total cholesterol,
    especially with high LDL and/or low HDL
Highly stressed personality ("type A" but ? constructive vs destructive
    stress)
Cardiopulmonary symptoms or signs
Abnormal resting or stress ECG (beware of false-positives) or pulmonary
    function tests
Abnormal hematologic, metabolic, or other blood or urine testing
Degree of motivation and ability to improve life-style

Other risk factors include family and/or personal history of heavy smoking and alcohol abuse, obesity, and poor diet quality and pattern. Notice the concept of diet quality and pattern, rather than just plain diet. It is beginning to be accepted, albeit a little grudgingly in cardiology, that the sedentary life-style is a true risk factor. I hope it will climb on the priority list in the next few years. Other risk factors include hypertension, prediabetic or established diabetic status, a highly compulsive striving personality called "type A," cardiopulmonary symptoms, abnormal resting or stress ECGs, abnormal pulmonary function tests, hematologic, metabolic, or other blood or urine tests, and finally, degree of motivation and ability to improve life-style. If a person is simply not motivated, especially after an educational effort, I view this as a risk factor.

LIFE-STYLE CHANGE

Having gone through history, examination, testing, and deciding what the risk factors are, laying the groundwork for a life-style change becomes a matter of first making sure your patient understands that the change must be permanent (Table 2-4). Dr Arnot has already pointed out some of the advantages of long-term training, but I am not talking about marathon running for the average patient. I am talking about adequate permanent, not temporary, exercise habits. The short-term goals and short-term approach, I find, generally do not work. Too many people are looking for magic and we have little magic in medicine.

Benefits

The many positive rewards that are commonly experienced when a poor life-style is improved, especially with proper diet and aerobic exercise, must be emphasized. Dr Arnot (Chapter 1) has already outlined the physiologic events that occur. It is exciting and interesting, but if you talk about fast-twitch and slow-twitch fibers to the average patient you have to be careful not to overwhelm him. Rather, I discuss the improved energy and sense of well-being, better stress-coping, and automatic eventual control of excess body fat.

24

Table 2-4
Laying the Groundwork for Life-style Change

1. **Essential** to get across the idea of permanent changes in life-style—acquiring new, regular, and lasting habits that are ultimately much more enjoyable. Shun the short-term goals—no such thing as magic!

2. **Emphasize** the many positive rewards commonly experienced when poor life-styles (and risk factors) are improved, especially with proper diet and enough aerobic exercise. These include:

   Improved energy and sense of well-being
   Better stress-coping (physical and mental)
   Automatic eventual control of excess body fat
   Apparent protection against coronary artery disease as measured by incidence of myocardial infarction
   Better control of hyperglycemia, often without medication
   Better control of systolic and diastolic hypertension, sometimes without medication
   Better quality of sleep (more restful)
   Better job performance
   Significantly improved self-image and pride accompanying superior fitness, loss of obesity, cessation of smoking, etc
   Vital importance of good example for one's children or youth groups, peers
   Significant reduction in number of upper respiratory tract infections and allergic rhinitis/asthma manifestations (in my experience)
   Significant improvement in depression and anxiety, often reducing need for medication
   Improved energy for extracurricular activities
   Significant reduction in long-term cost of medical care, as unnecessary illness is prevented or deferred
   Greater longevity with good quality of life?

3. **Avoid** scare tactics—the identified risk factors should be presented in a matter-of-fact manner, simply as items of important information to help an intelligent person make a commitment to a life-style change

4. **Understanding** takes teaching, which takes time, but it begets willingness to make a commitment—after that, it is just organization

In my practice we de-emphasize weight and we ask our patients not to concentrate on it. After all, the scale is measuring not just fat, but also muscle, bone, and fluid. It is a common and tragic mistake to think that the minute the scale says you have gained weight, you have gained fat. Actually, people doing everything right, getting into really good aerobic exercise condition, and eating with proper quality and pattern will gain some weight, but will have lost excess body fat. The muscle mass increase simply adds to the weight. So, if you point this out and have people shun these multitudes of short-term and really crazy things they do to lose fat, then you are doing them an enormous favor. The point has to be stressed over and over again because we are all so conditioned to think in terms only of the special short-term fat loss.

Other benefits are the apparent protection against coronary artery disease as measured by incidence of myocardial infarction, and better control of hyperglycemia, often without medication, as muscles are shown to have an increased sensitivity to insulin.[2] Systolic and diastolic hypertension control is improved as is the quality of sleep. Job performance is enhanced and so is self-image.

Aerobic exercise of itself is useful in helping to reduce addictive behavior. Many people who have not been able to cut down on alcohol, quit smoking, or have trouble with compulsive eating, find the ability after starting an aerobic exercise program. It is vitally important to set a good example for children and youth groups. A point I often make to my patients is do not forget that our children and the kids we work with are going to be controlling us in the last 25 years of our lives. You have to ask yourself, considering the expanding areas of control of our senior citizens' lives, "Whom do you want in those jobs 35 to 40 years from now?"

A significant reduction in the number of cold and allergic rhinitis symptoms in my experience has been exciting. I hear patients remark so often on an annual return engagement that they have not had a cold in the past year, where they always used to. I cannot prove its significance, but I hear it much too often for it to be accidental. Significant improvement in depression and anxiety states is also seen. The use of aerobic exercise is today frequently described in the psychiatric literature and is generating a lot of excitement in that field. There is also improved energy for extra-curricular activities.

It is pleasing to see the number of my patients who used to go home and crash in front of the TV who are now energized and involved in various community tasks and activities. In other words, we can do a great deal not only at the personal and family level but also at the community level if we have the energy to do so. Finally, I think significant reductions can occur in the long-term cost of medical care, as unnecessary illness is prevented or deferred. A recent study in *Medical World News* made this very point.[3] A group of patients with fit life-styles was compared against a group with more typical sedentary and unfit life-styles. Over a four-year period there was a more than $4000 difference in costs of hospital and office expenses between these two groups. That is of great interest to us where there is so much governmental effort to address the cost of medical care in what may turn out to be a very short-sighted way. This message needs to be carried loud and clear to our legislators: namely, that we would much rather have long-range programs encouraging health and fitness as opposed to more government- controlled crisis-oriented care.

Finally, the question of greater longevity with good quality of life is raised by improving cardiovascular mortality. Too many of us die too young from coronary artery disease. If it is possible to protect against this—and there is good evidence to say we can—then we may indeed have both more years and a better quality of life.

Motivation

The above are the subjects that I like to bring up to my patients. They emphasize the positive rather than scare tactics. An intelligent person who is told of his problems and the benefits that can result from a life-style change has the background to do three very important things. He can understand the need for change. A person must know what is going on and why. Second, armed with this information hopefully he can make a commitment to a life-style change provided he has been given the tools with which to make these changes. Third, taking this approach—emphasizing understanding and having the patient build a commitment—the change boils down very simply to a matter of organization and scheduling. Such terms as "self-discipline" and "willpower" should be avoided as they sometimes are used as an excuse not to change.

On selecting options for a life-style change (Table 2-5), I will not say much about smoking because it is self-explanatory. It simply has to stop. It is an extremely dangerous problem. The risks are not only pulmonary (cancer, emphysema, etc) but cardiovascular mortality is also influenced. I find it very useful to point out, especially to parents of small children, that their behavior influences their children's. Thus if they smoke there is a greater chance their children will become smokers in later life. We also know that children who grow up with someone smoking in the family have a higher incidence of upper respiratory infections and allergies. If something a parent is doing technically harms a child we have a term for it: child abuse. I find that often jolts people who are smokers; I have been able to reach smokers with this concept. If they have small children the thought that they could actually be harming their kids may move them where what they are doing to themselves may not.

Shunning special calorie-counting or otherwise restricted diets is very important unless restrictions are needed for medical purposes. The quality and pattern of eating is enormously important. If you are talking about permanent life-style changes then the short-term solution, the special diet, should be avoided. If you can teach a person to eat a solid breakfast of high quality, a light lunch, and a moderate supper, you are going a long way not only toward giving them a better quality of performance during the day mentally and physically, but also supporting a good exercise program.

One of the interesting phenomena with aerobic exercise, almost universally, has been that many people notice a drop-off in appetite for the excesses. I certainly did, and I have seen it in the great majority of my patients. Analogies are very useful and I liken the good breakfast to simply putting gas in the tank of a

Table 2-5
Selecting Options for a Life-style Change

1. **Stop** smoking!!!

2. **Shun** special calorie-counting or otherwise restricted diets; teach proper quality and pattern of eating (solid breakfast—never skipped, light lunch, moderate supper)

3. **Emphasize** the enormous variety that is available within the above pattern, still with good quality (the many high-fiber cereals with whole and cracked grains, fruits, lean meats, juices, milk, fresh vegetables, large salads particularly as a main course at supper)

4. **No** focusing on weight!! Excess fat always disappears if a proper and permanent diet quality and pattern are accompanied by solid levels of aerobic exercise

5. **Explain** aerobic exercise in practical terms (nonintermittent activity generating 75% to 80% age-adjusted maximal heart rate for progressively longer periods as good condition is achieved; new standard of 2000 kcal/week approximately equals three hours at this heart rate)

6. **Help** patient pick whatever truly aerobic exercise form seems most enjoyable, but also most practical and safe. Jogging is the least expensive and most efficient for many, but other options include: swimming, cross-country skiing, bicycling, snowshoeing, rowing, ice skating, roller skating, roller skiing, fast walking, walk-jogging, or nonstop squash, racquetball, or handball

---

very fine car. I will mention to a patient that if he had a Mercedes or Rolls Royce and were going to take a long trip somewhere, he would fill the gas tank first.

The enormous variety that is available within the above pattern must be emphasized also. The average supermarket can provide good nutrition. In general have a patient buy high-fiber cereals with whole or cracked grain, good quality breads, fruits, lean meats, low-fat milk, and fresh vegetables. I particularly emphasize eating large salads at supper because it is the problem meal in our society—much too large and full of too many things that have the metabolism struggling all night, thus making breakfast a much more difficult proposition. Having patients (particularly breakfast-skippers) eat only salads, at least for a while, as their dinner greatly reduces calories while providing excellent nutrition. Eating a good breakfast then becomes easier as one is hungrier by morning.

Again I emphasize to have people not focus on weight. With proper diet and exercise excess body fat will disappear. How long this takes will depend on how much exercise a person is able to do and how well they progress. The concept of a permanent life-style change helps and when the fat is going and people see it disappearing, they become more motivated as they experience the pride of achievement.

Society at large is only barely beginning to be aware of what aerobic exercise really is and unfortunately there are misunderstandings. There are a lot of people that roll around with big muscles and are fairly trim whom the public regards as being in superb condition. And, indeed they may be isometrically in excellent condition, but the cardiovascular system may not have been well trained at all. It is not uncommon to find some of these gentlemen in their forties and fifties either dead on arrival in the emergency room or staring in bewilderment at the coronary care unit ceiling after a heart attack. Thus the concept of aerobic exercise where the heart rate gets up to 70% to 80% of age-adjusted maximal rates, for progressively longer periods as good condition improves, is stressed. We encourage this aerobic exercise to minimally expend 2000 kcal per week, which translates into about three hours. For a runner it is relatively easy, you can approximate 100 kcal per mile and go from there. Help a patient pick whatever aerobic exercise form seems to be most enjoyable, practical, and safe.

Implementation

Since I run, I am called the "jogging doctor." But I find sometimes that I have to counteract this for some people for whom jogging is either of no interest or not suitable. There are many, many other aerobic sports. Any sport that is nonintermittent and causes a relatively high heart rate can be suggested. Options are listed in Table 2-5. Swimming, running, and cross-country skiing are at the very top of the energy expenditure list. Others include bicycling, snowshoeing, rowing, ice skating, roller skating, roller skiing, fast walking, walk-jogging, nonstop squash, racquetball, handball, and aerobic dancing.

At the end of a complete history and physical examination, you should know your patient pretty well, ie, what he or she likes, does, would like to do, and whether he is going to be able to move ahead with this, and at what pace. The best and most important way of getting going with all these changes is to try to do them simultaneously (Table 2-6). You will find people very often saying, "Let's see, this sounds like a lot. I would rather quit smoking and kind of wait on the other things or maybe I'll do some exercise but I'm not so sure about the diet or the smoking." I have found that if a person is going to make a life-style change and make a commitment to it, these activities support each other.

Safety should be emphasized. This is a new area; there are a number of people within and without the profession, who write articles every day that point out the dangers, real and imagined. It is necessary that the patient understand that a gradual progression is essential in any aerobic exercise program, and particularly in jogging, which has the highest injury rate. Be sure with any of these exercises that the patient understands proper warm-up, especially stretching exercises, which are important for preventing injury. I point out to people trying to learn, especially runners, to do distance first, rather than worrying about pace. Too many people spend too much time thinking about what they did the day before or what their neighbor is doing. Patients must understand this is their own individual program and it is much more important to arrive at good distances safely and enjoyably than it is to go too hard, too fast, and get hurt en route. A proper cool-off period must also be emphasized.

Reinforcement

The teaching function is important if a person is going to achieve a life-style change successfully. People must come back for follow-up visits; it is as simple as that. You cannot launch a boat, slide it down the way, break a bottle of champagne over it,

Table 2-6
Implementing Life-style Changes

1. **Urge** all necessary changes be begun and continued more or less simultaneously—they support each other!

2. **Emphasize** the absolute necessity for regularity; this is the organization and scheduling part (not "self-discipline" or "willpower"—these terms are used as cop-outs!).

3. **Be sure** your patient knows the importance of proper warm-up (especially stretching exercises), gradual progression of pace (this is endurance conditioning, and learning to do distance/time first and faster paces later is important), and proper cool-off.

4. **Outline** the teaching function (like any other adult education course) of follow-up visits to ensure safe and effective progress, and insist upon them; point out the patient's investment of time and money in self; use analogies—launching a boat, learning to fly an airplane, tuning up and maintaining a fine car, etc.

5. **Ask** for a well-maintained exercise record to assess regularity, degree and rate of progress, and whether or not the patient is pushing too hard or fast.

6. **Reinforce** any progress (the means are simple, but life-style change itself is tough for many), and try to be non-judgmental about any failures. Locate the obstacle to progress if possible and try to help the patient find a way around it.

7. **Set** a good personal example! Patients are much impressed if their own doctor is a jogger or vigorous regular aerobic exerciser of any type. Practicing what we preach seems to help.

8. **Graduate** your successful patient from regular follow-up (assuming it is not needed for other medical problems) when you have ascertained that he is self-sustaining at a good aerobic level—I use 2000 kcal/week—and enjoying it, without overuse symptoms or other exercise-related problems. Then help keep him there by as-needed visits if illness or injury intervenes, or annual examinations by mutual agreement.

say good bye, good luck, see you in a year: the boat still has to be steered. I have found, not entirely to my surprise, that people do not like to see doctors. People get a mixed message if told, "gee, you are in excellent health, come back and see me." A lot of people, because of conditioning, see a doctor only when sick, and do not come back for follow-up. The original motivation and excitement dwindle, interruptions occur, and the life-style change gets nowhere. Today I point out that even if a person has no medical problems, the need exists to be followed up at regular intervals. Again analogies are useful, such as tuning or maintaining a fine car; what finer machine could you have than your biological one? Keeping it at least at minimal maintenance is the goal.

Keeping a well-maintained exercise record is very important in the training stages. The instructor really needs to be sure exactly what is going on to avoid an overuse problem. The record should include a daily account of the type, duration, and intensity of primary exercise pursued. Any warm-up or cool-off exercises as well as duration and type of any nonrecreational exercise, ie, mowing the lawn, shoveling snow, vacuuming the house, etc, should also be listed.

Reinforcing progress is vital as is praising anything a patient is doing that is a step in the right direction, even if it is not up to the standards that have originally been outlined. It is a tricky business that can be discouraging at first and follow-up visits serve as reinforcement. Being nonjudgmental about failures is also important because many people who are trying to achieve and are not having good luck feel guilty. Here it is best to say "let's find what the problem is and see if we can work our way around the obstacle."

A personal example is important. The physician, nurse, physical therapist—anyone who is working with a patient— should do some aerobics with regularity. It improves teaching effectiveness to practice what you preach. Many patients ask in a somewhat challenging manner if I run or exercise, etc. I would feel awfully uncomfortable if I could not answer positively.

Graduating the successful patient from regular follow-up is important. We use the 2000 kcal goal, a point where you can return to the more standard doctor-patient relationship but at a much better level.

REFERENCES

1. Paffenbarger, R.S., Wing, A.L., and Hyde, R.T. Physical activity and an index of heart attack risk in college alumni. *Am J Epidemiol.* 108:161–175, 1978.

2. Soman, V.R., Kovisto, V.A., Deibert, D., et al. Increased insulin sensitivity and insulin binding to monocytes after physical training. *N Engl J Med.* 301:1200–1204, 1979.

3. *Medical World News.* Keeping fit holds medical bills down, says Purdue study. 12(25):16, 1978.

3 Corporate Physical Fitness—the Rewards to Industry and Society

Robert Burns Arnot, MD

The summer of 1979, New England Running *was the beneficiary of an outstanding article on Corporate Physical Fitness by the author of this chapter. A marathoner, competitive cyclist, and cross-country skier of near Olympic caliber himself, Dr Arnot will tell us why it is good business for industry to "shape up."*

The concept of corporate fitness has its origins in the 19th century at the Institute for Work Physiology in Stockholm, Sweden. Work physiology evolved as an outgrowth of social concern for conditions at the place of labor. Foremost, it sought "to make it possible for the individual to do his job without undue fatigue and still be able to enjoy his leisure time," to quote work physiologist Per-Olaf Astrand.[1] With automation, many industrial employees were relieved of any true physical exertion; physical labor virtually disappeared from agrarian, service, and professional ranks.

It was with the discovery of oxygen itself by Lavoisier over two hundred years ago that interest in work physiology was born. The small institute in Sweden has heralded most of the major discoveries in exercise physiology in the last hundred years.

It was in the 19th century that investigators first looked scientifically at what employees did at their place of work. The motivating force was not the health of the worker, but how much effort could be extracted from him. It was determined that 45% of maximum oxygen consumption was all that an individual could sustain for eight or more hours a day and still return home in a functional status for his family and be capable of rising the next morning for a similar work effort. The Scandinavians were, thus, able to prescribe maximal work loads for workers at various jobs.

Today, almost as novel, work physiology reappears to introduce "work" to industry in the form of exercise, beginning with the highest corporate ranks. Now, as then, the focus is cardiopulmonary performance and muscular fatigue. Machines, which once replaced the laborer, are brought again to the workplace, this time bringing the laborer back to "work."

The impetus behind this situation is clear: as the late John Knowles, former Chief of Massachusetts General Hospital and President of the Rockefeller Foundation said often, "The next big advance in modern medicine will be in what the patient can do for himself."

Not only does modern medicine hold little hope of startling breakthroughs, but, in fact, all of cardiovascular and transplant surgery, antibiotics, and intensive care medicine—much of the physician's armamentarium—contributed little to increase life expectancy during the greatest development years of modern medicine, 1920 to 1970. Only with control of high blood pressure, decreased alcohol consumption, anti-smoking campaigns, and better diet and fitness did life expectancy rise from 1970 to the present.

The President's Council on Physical Fitness and Sports reports that 13 cents of every federal dollar is spent on health care; less than 2% of this is spent on prevention. The significance of these figures increases in light of the 700,000 yearly deaths from heart disease alone. The Council estimates that 115,000 premature deaths would be avoided every year if each adult over 30 would walk one mile per day.

A nationwide Lou Harris Poll,[2] sponsored by Perrier, documents that those who expend at least 1500 calories a week in exercise feel better in general and have a more positive outlook on life. They sleep better, are better able to deal with pressure, are more assertive, think more creatively, believe that they will live longer, and have a better self-image. By no small coincidence, epidemiologist Ralph Paffenbarger et al, in a long-term study of 17,000 Harvard graduates, indicated that expending 2000 kcal, or four hours of weekly jogging at 5.5 miles per hour, will result in a 64% statistical chance of not having a heart attack.[3] This applies not only to the experienced competitor, but to the individual who begins and maintains that level of fitness later in life as well.

The fitness claim is further expanded by the California Health Department's Human Population Library estimates of adding 11 years to the life expectancy of men and 7 to that of women through optimizing living habits.

Corporate Response

The corporate response to this emerging fitness consciousness has been to finance million-dollar programs, no longer for key executives alone, but for larger employee groups. Motives remain unclear, however, when machine- and facility-oriented programs—appealing to the media and the public at large—are instituted to gain broad exposure to corporate "good guys" ostensibly saying, "your company cares about your well-being."

The expertise, the precise, brilliantly conceived professional effort behind the fitness movement, pales against the backdrop of new capital acquisition and product-line management strategy. Yet, industrial chiefs, mystified by a profession and science to which they have had little exposure, are willing to accept vague generalities regarding exercise: it is good for you, you may live longer, it will hold the line on employee benefits, decrease absenteeism, and increase morale and productivity. The same board of directors that heavily invests in various consulting services to shape fiscal and public policy finds itself having built an expensive health spa, country club, or the like, which some would say is merely a diversion at best.

Exercise, on an upswing and highly visible, is chosen hopefully as a powerful stimulus for employees to examine personal habits that affect general health, and hence, their work performance. Is it, though, a new and expected employee benefit?

When, in fact, have you seen a truck driver jogging at a truck stop or a janitor spending his lunch break on the company's racquetball court? Several hundred firms now have fitness programs, yet only 30 allow all employees to participate. Few companies can afford not to be elitist given the great facility costs of their programs, further increased if staffing includes a physiologist, physical therapist, or cardiologist. Concurrently, one finds the glittering company pool, massive weight training stations, and designer-decorated calisthenic rooms, often unused in a structured approach as programs lack rigorously defined objectives.

Suggestions

Less expensive and perhaps more effective for many companies might be imposed dietary restriction, no smoke/drink policies, personnel screening and counselling for bad health habits, or hiring policies restricting employment to those who take care of themselves. Large corporations, some with the income and population of a small country, might adopt the attitude assumed by the Royal College of Surgeons several years ago: our health care system should not have to pay for your excesses. With spiraling health care costs, fitness should be regarded as a national asset, not a burden.

In a country where millions are spent on scientific esoterica at the ocean's floor and in outer space, it appears ludicrous that we are not similarly engaged in a major scientific and management effort aimed at documenting and implementing such a universal form of preventive medicine as physical fitness. Instead, we rely on the current, largely piecemeal, media-oriented approach.

The task of physicians, moreover, is often too simplistic. "Don't overdo it," or "Start out slowly," are often given as instructions with no sense of pace or quality of exercise. The greatest single deterrent to good regular exercise is a lack of detailed knowledge. The situation is made little better by irresponsible journalism stating that "jogging will kill you," or the like. It is illustrative that bowling is considered sufficient conditioning for fitness by one-third of the American populace.

Who is in shape? Insurance companies such as the innovative Occidental Life of North Carolina believe that long-distance runners, joggers, swimmers, and bicyclists are; marathoners are not even required to submit to a medical exam. "Now your exercise can pay off in CASH SAVINGS even though you may not be a professional," reads one of their brochures offering to adjust your insurance rate to reflect your good health. Certainly the rate cutbacks in health and life insurance premiums benefit employee, insurer, and employer.

Unlike socialist countries, Americans have been largely self-motivated, without a structured program. Government, industry, and commercial sponsors have been unable to put labels on what people do for themselves. The real irony is that those of us considered most fit, at least for risk of heart attack, are serious runners—and this includes the President. Few of this group have ever seen the inside of a plushly carpeted health spa or rely on equipment more expensive than good shoes, education more costly than *New England Running,* or professional advice beyond Bill Rodgers' free Saturday Clinics. The fittest Americans have few accouterments of their pursuit.

For the majority of those who are serious about their level of fitness, nothing could be more boring or short-lived than stationary exercise bicycles, the treadmill, or indoor minitrack. (These, in fact, are usually regarded as facilitating recovery from injury and/or surgery, not as a perennial means of maintaining fitness.) While CBS may own sprawling health spas, the majority of us are still fighting for the acceptability of exercise at work: time out to run before dark, a safe place to run during lunch hour, showers, bike racks, lockers, changing facilities, laundry service, and subsidies for the local YMCA or nearby pool are legitimate concerns. The more real problems for employees in both business and government involve the logistics and scheduling of exercise regimens created by those individuals for themselves.

And what about corporations that do not have fitness programs? The largest life insurance company in New England, for instance, has yet to make a decision: "Is it safe?" ask their trustees. Certainly the short-term training studies of published conscientious researchers show dramatic effects, but how safe is it to recommend similar programs to the unwatched masses of a large firm?

As a bottom line, one must protect the end organ and the tools used to train it:

1. If, in fact, a well-trained heart is what we want, it should be protected against high-pressure work loads, as well as excessive adrenaline and lactic acid buildup precipitated by severe exertion. With proper training, pressure load on the heart, levels of lactic acid, and adrenaline are lower at high work loads.

2. The muscles and their supporting structures are the tools used to develop the heart. Thus, great care must also be taken to acknowledge the long development time of the muscles. Seventy-one-year-old John Kelley, for example, often recommends no running at all in the first months of a fitness program (personal communication). By perfecting these tools, the exercise is safer and the conditioning longer-lived.

The conceptual stages of any program must include rigorously defined objectives. Aside from the peripheral health spa approach, these objectives are embodied in *performance,* which can be strictly defined, marked, and followed, thus demonstrating the efficacy of exercise rather than awaiting a nebulous final word on increasing longevity. It is, after all, how *well* one lives, not how *long,* that concerns most of us. Performance can be subjectively assessed, objectively measured. The quantity of exercise that will produce certain physiologic effects associated with a statistical guarantee of protection against heart attacks is known.

The minute measurement of muscle cell chemistry, heart biophysics, and nervous control of movement is commonplace in top US and European human performance laboratories. With the proper sample size, large firms can statistically validate fitness and its relation to absenteeism, productivity, and insurance premiums. They can also legitimately document each physiologic mechanism, thus tailoring training to the specific needs of employees whether technician, ditchdigger, or chief executive officer. It is likewise important to note that this undertaking, by occupation, allows further application to many thousands of other people. Only one study, another by Paffenbarger et al with longshoremen, indicates the intensity of exercise needed for prevention of heart attacks.[3] This intensity-duration-frequency formula goes well beyond quantity-oriented aerobics to implicate precise mechanisms of change in the body.

The formulas derived may be enacted through individualization for jobs: aerobic training for the longshoreman, greater walking pace for the night watchman, increased volume of exercise for calorie-plagued cafeteria workers, stretching for the executive marathoner. With careful conceptual planning, the needs of employee classes may be determined and validated. Cardiovascular, pulmonary, and muscular performance may judge the physical, while the subjective benefits may be measured by advanced psychological tests as well as on-the-job performance—improvement in motor and/or interactive skills, increased sales quotas.

Those companies and individuals who have embarked upon the corporate fitness course are to be heartily congratulated. They deserve all of the credit given them when so many other enterprises, scientists, and physicians are unwilling to make a commitment at all.

Industry is where fitness is happening as an organized entity, as recognized by the President's Council on Physical Fitness and Sports. The next generation is learning this new physical education in the classroom; the rest of us rely on ourselves or our employers. It has become their responsibility to proceed with well-defined principles to create and support fitness programs geared to the needs and wants of their employees, and, using scientific guidelines, to document the efficacy of their programs.

The most sophisticated country on earth, being given its panacea, now requires the scientific and public information to make it work simply and universally.

REFERENCES

1. Astrand, P.O., and Rodahl, K. *Textbook of Work Physiology.* New York: McGraw-Hill, 1977.

2. *The Perrier Study: Fitness in America.* New York: The Perrier Corporation, 1979.

3. Paffenbarger, R.S., Wing, A.L., and Hyde, R.T. Physical activity and an index of heart attack risk in college alumni. *Am J Epidemiol.* 108:161–175, 1978.

4 Nutrition and Endurance Exercise— Facts, Myths, Speculations

Robert C. Cantu, MD

As fitness has become a popular topic, media hype and often less-than-benevolent promotion has become a part of the scene. Unfortunately, considerable inaccurate information has crossed our TV screens and padded newspapers and magazines. I can remember myself in 1966/1967 entering long-distance races where the prize, with the exception of the winner, was a cup of coffee and doughnuts. Our entry fee was a quarter or half-dollar maximum. Now, the entry fees exceed $5.00, you receive a 98¢ T-shirt, and the sponsors make money. Perhaps in no area have more half-truths, myths, and just plain erroneous information been dispersed than in nutrition, the subject of this chapter.

It goes without saying that a close relationship exists between diet, nutrition, and physical exercise. First, individuals who exercise regularly make heavy demands upon their body's reserves of fluid and energy. One must be aware of the special dietary and nutritional needs created as a result of their exercise program. The ordinary diet will need to be supplemented and adjusted if one is to realize the maximum benefit from an exercise program. Before discussing the special dietary requirements of exercise, a few basic comments about general dietary objectives for Americans will be presented.

The recent McGovern Committee that studied American dietary habits concluded that Americans *eat too much and eat the wrong things.* They consume too much meat, saturated fat, cholesterol, sugar, and salt. At the same time, they do not eat enough fruit, grain—especially whole grain products—vegetables, and unsaturated fat. The Committee urged American leaders to educate the public to increase its consumption of fruits, vegetables, and whole grain cereals, and to sharply reduce its intake of fat and sugar.

The suggestions of the Committee, although physiologically sound, will not be easily implemented in this country. They run counter to obvious ethnic and cultural patterns of eating that are longstanding. Implementation may also cause heavy financial losses to major food producers and manufacturers who control food advertising, especially advertising of sugar-laden cereals that appeal to children. These companies may not welcome an attempt to change the financially successful "sugared" status quo.

Despite the expected resistance from cultural markets and big business, the recommended dietary changes will ultimately be realized. Today, Americans are more fitness-conscious than ever before and the enthusiasm is far from cresting. More Americans today are pursuing strenuous physical exercise than ever before. Dietary lunacy is a necessary by-product of such concern for one's physical well-being. The old adage that you are what you eat is poignantly pertinent today.

LOSING WEIGHT THROUGH DIET AND EXERCISE

Body weight is lost when one or more of the body's substances is decreased, thus reducing total body mass. Short-term weight loss can be effected by loss of water, fat, protein, or glycogen. Such weight loss occurs frequently during periods of strenuous exercise, as will be discussed below. Longer-term weight loss also depletes minerals from the bone and soft tissues of the body. Actually, weight loss is a simple biologic process that is related to the protein, glycogen, and water that exist in the body. Every gram of protein or glycogen has coupled with it approximately 3 to 4 gm of water. When a deficit of protein or glycogen occurs, there follows necessarily water loss as well. Presently, it is not established that there is any water loss when triglycerides are mobilized from adipose cells.

Until recently, it was thought that on average, 1 lb (0.45 kg) of body weight loss corresponded to the burning of about 3500 kcal. This figure was derived from a value that suggested that 98% of the calories burned were derived from body fat. Studies now show that during the first several weeks of dietary restriction, weight loss is far in excess of the caloric deficit and reflects primarily water loss. Much of this initial water loss is due to a poorly understood diuresis that occurs with loss of sodium and water. However, the other is the obligatory water loss that accompanies the depletion of body glycogen stores. Later in a caloric restriction diet, the water diuresis stops entirely and in some instances a water gain can occur while net losses of fat and protein continue.

It is of interest to note that different diets can produce an acceleration of weight loss due to greater water loss. For instance, a diet low in carbohydrate, the extreme being a fast, will cause a greater water diuresis and more precipitous weight loss. During a prolonged partial, or total, caloric restriction, the body gradually adapts by conserving protein and water and increasingly burning fat to make up the energy deficit. Studies show[1] that obese individuals accomplish this adaptation more rapidly than lean people. However, the key finding is that the body's fat loss is essentially proportional to its energy deficit. So, in the end, the type of diet is relatively unimportant. What ultimately determines fat loss is the degree of caloric deprivation. Because of this, most nutritionists now recommend a balanced diet that combines smaller portions of the basic foods with a reduction or elimination of refined sugars and desserts. Such a diet not only accomplishes weight reduction, but also instills eating habits that promote the maintenance of desired weight.

As surely as the sun rises and sets, there will always be one more diet that promises quick weight loss without effort. The latest fad is the "Last Chance Diet" or "Protein-Supplemented Fasting," an essentially no-carbohydrate diet that supplies nutrition by a mixture of liquid proteins, vitamins, and minerals. The promoters of Last Chance Diet claim that when protein is provided in the diet, the body does not use its own protein, and thus minimizes muscle waste and the depletion of body protein stores. But is this really so? Not according to an article published in *The New England Journal of Medicine* that recently reported "although some consider a low-calorie diet consisting entirely of protein to be uniquely advantageous in preserving body nitrogen, it has yet to be demonstrated convincingly that protein alone is more effective in this regard than an isocaloric mixture of protein and carbohydrate."[1] Whenever carbohydrate intake is severely restricted as it is in the Last Chance Diet, fat is mobilized and rapid mobilization of fat may cause serious side effects including liver damage. Also, low potassium levels may result, and even cardiac arrhythmia deaths have been attributed to this diet. The chemical imbalance created by the loss of salt, water, and other minerals may lead to weakness, faintness, and other side effects. Even more tragic—because these diets do not encourage the proper way of eating—only one-third of those who follow them are able to keep fat off 18 months after abandoning them.

Influence of Diet and Exercise on Cholesterol, Cardiovascular Disease, and Atherosclerosis

The knowledge acquired over the past few decades about cholesterol, cardiovascular disease, and atherosclerosis indicates that a carefully combined program of diet and exercise can greatly retard these diseases. Arteriosclerosis is a process by which the walls of our body's vessels become infiltrated with fat, which in time calcifies and forms plaques that can occlude an artery. It is seldom localized. When it develops in a major vessel to the brain or lower extremities, for example, there is nearly always similar impairment of the coronary arteries of the heart. In fact, the major cause of death in patients following surgery for localized atherosclerosis is heart attack.[2]

The precise mechanism by which cholesterol is deposited in the walls of arteries and an advanced plaque evolves is still being unraveled. It is apparent, though, that multiple defects in cellular cholesterol metabolism, as well as smooth muscle cell proliferation, are involved. While the means by which even normal cells are proliferated and build up cholesterol remain an enigma, certain correlations regarding cholesterol are apparent.

Blood contains two classes of fats that are essential to life: cholesterol and triglycerides. Elevated levels of cholesterol and/or triglycerides are associated with accelerated atherosclerosis and increased probability of heart attack. Of the multiple factors that influence the blood levels of these fats, diet, heredity, and exercise are the most important. A reduction in blood triglycerides and cholesterol occurs with exercise and with a diet low in saturated fats.

Cholesterol is transported by protein compounds called lipoproteins. Recent investigations have shown that the total level of cholesterol is of less importance than the ratio of high-density lipoprotein (HDL) to low-density lipoprotein (LDL). Low-density lipoproteins are the harmful transport vehicles that carry cholesterol into the tissues and enhance the buildup of fatty atherosclerotic plaques. Conversely, high-density lipoproteins are capable of transporting cholesterol out of arteries and tissues and into the liver where it is broken down and eliminated. A high level of HDL to LDL correlates with a low risk for atherosclerosis and heart disease. Vigorous sustained exercise will raise high-density lipoprotein levels and lower low-density lipoprotein levels. A diet low in saturated fats will achieve the same result. Triglycerides are also lowered by exercise and correlate with the HDL to LDL ratio. Elevated triglyceride levels are seen with increased levels of low-density lipoprotein, while normal or low triglyceride levels are seen with elevated high-density lipoprotein levels.

Coffee, Alcohol, and Physical Exercise

A question that inevitably arises in the minds of those involved in a total exercise program is, "Must I stop using coffee and alcohol?" There is much misinformation about the effects of these two drugs. Several reports, for example, have suggested that moderate to heavy coffee drinking (6 to 10 cups daily) may predispose to heart attack. More recent studies,[3] however, show that coffee ingestion by itself is not harmful. These earlier reports failed to account for the fact that many coffee drinkers are also cigarette smokers, a practice that does predispose to heart attack, emphysema, and cancer. When cigarette smoking was taken into account, no increased incidence of heart attack was found in coffee drinkers.

Also contrary to earlier investigations, scientists now believe that moderate alcohol consumption, especially beer, is not harmful and indeed appears to protect the heart. One study,[3] which covered a six-year period, reported that "moderate beer drinkers" had only half the incidence of heart attack as those who totally abstained. It is still unclear whether alcohol itself has some protective value, or whether the teetotaler represents a rigid personality type that may predispose to heart attack. Beer has long been a favorite thirst quencher for many distance runners, and it is now very popular as a replacement solution during the long-distance runs including marathons. Indeed, beer has been credited with keeping the kidneys functioning during endurance exercise by blocking antidiuretic hormone (ADH) secretion and, thus, preventing kidney stones and hematuria from bruising the bladder. It has a high potassium and sodium ratio (5:1), thus is a safe sweat replacement preventing hypokalemia. It also replaces silicon and raises the level of high-density lipoproteins. While there is no proof of improved performance from beer drinkers, it does appear that some discomfort may be alleviated.

One caution concerning alcohol consumption is its high caloric content of 7 calories per gram. Only fat with 9 calories per gram has more by comparison (protein and carbohydrates each contain only 4 calories per gram). Anyone dieting should be informed about the high caloric content of alcohol and avoid its use. All of us should be aware that excessive alcohol intake may cause direct toxic damage to the liver and in some cases to the heart as well. This is true even with an adequate diet. The old belief that cirrhosis of the liver develops primarily in people who drink heavily and eat poorly is myth, not fact. Recent studies[4] show that an average-size person who drinks one-half bottle of 86 proof beverage per day for 25 years has a 50% chance of developing cirrhosis of the liver regardless of the diet. Today in the United States, there are an estimated 10 million plus alcoholics, and in urban areas cirrhosis of the liver is the third major cause of death between the ages of 25 and 65 years. Therefore, while moderate alcohol consumption, especially beer, is certainly not harmful and may even protect the heart, heavy drinking is very hazardous and poisons the brain, heart, and liver. Recent investigations have prompted a warning from the Surgeon General that cancer has been linked to heavy alcohol consumption.

VITAMINS—FACTS, FANCIES, AND MYTHS

For those following a strenuous daily exercise program, a knowledge of vitamins is absolutely essential since there may be a special need for vitamin supplements to achieve maximum benefit from exercise.

No human, indeed no mammal, can be maintained on an exclusive diet of protein, carbohydrate, fat, and minerals. Additional factors present in natural foods are required in minute amounts (Table 4-1). These organic substances, vitamins, function as chemical regulators and are necessary for growth and the maintenance of life. There are 14 known vitamins and they divide into two basic groups: those soluble in fat (vitamins A, D, E, and K), and those soluble in water (vitamin C and the B complex vitamins). Normally, a varied diet contains more than enough of these required vitamins. As they do not contribute to body structure and are not a direct source of body energy, even the most active athlete needs little more than does the sedentary individual.

It has only been since the advent of the industrial revolution, urbanization, and sea travel, that many people have not had access to a varied farm diet of recently harvested foodstuffs, and that vitamin deficiencies have been known. Sailors who spent months at sea without fruit or green vegetables developed scurvy from a lack of vitamin C. Impoverished Southeast Asians whose diets are restricted to polished rice develop vitamin B deficiencies, and infants in crowded European slums, deprived of adequate sunlight, develop rickets from a deficiency of vitamin D.

49

Table 4-1
Recommended Daily Allowances of Vitamins (United States)

Vitamin	Infants and children up to 4 years	Children 4 years to adults
Vitamin A	2500 IU	5000 IU
Thiamine (B_1)	0.7 mg	1.5 mg
Riboflavin (B_2)	0.8 mg	1.7 mg
Vitamin B_6	0.7 mg	2 mg
Vitamin B_{12}	3 mg	6 mg
Folacin (Bc)	0.2 mg	0.4 mg
Biotin	0.15 mg	0.3 mg
Niacin	9 mg	20 mg
Pantothenic acid	5 mg	10 mg
Ascorbic acid (C)	40 mg	60 mg
Vitamin D	400 IU	400 IU
Vitamin E	10 IU	30 IU

One man who has contributed much to our modern understanding of vitamin deficiency is Professor Victor Herbert. Professor Herbert states succinctly that "the sole unequivocal indication for vitamin therapy is vitamin deficiency."[5] He discusses six ways in which vitamin deficiency develops: inadequate ingestion, absorption, or utilization; and increased destruction, excretion, or requirement. Of the six possible causes of vitamin deficiency that Herbert cites, inadequate ingestion is the only indication for dietary vitamin supplementation.

The fat soluble vitamins (A, D, E, and K) are stored in the liver and adipose tissue. Deficiencies develop only after months or years of inadequate intake, and excessive intake will cause abnormal accumulations and can produce toxic side effects. The water soluble vitamins are not stored in the body and must be constantly replenished in the diet. Deficiencies can develop in weeks, and when excessive amounts are ingested, the excess is excreted in the urine avoiding toxic accumulations.

Except during periods of extra nutrient demand such as pregnancy, lactation, or prolonged illness, the AMA does not recommend vitamin supplementation. Today, however, the use of multivitamin preparations is commonplace. This is not harmful so long as fat soluble vitamins are not taken in excess. The essential foodstuffs can usually come from our diet and need not be found in any vitamin bottle. These "essential" nutrients, ie, those which cannot be manufactured by the body, include water, sources of energy (primarily carbohydrates), nine amino acid building blocks of proteins, one fatty acid, a number of mineral elements, and vitamins. Only a diet including a selection from a wide variety of foods will ensure adequate essential nutrient intake.

Vitamins in Deficiency States

The American Medical Association advises that the use of vitamin preparations as dietary supplements ought to be restricted to specific instances of deficiency; then, only the deficient vitamins in therapeutic amounts should be prescribed along with measures to correct any dietary inadequacies. Some common medical conditions requiring vitamin therapy include the malabsorption syndromes (tropical sprue and celiac disease) where vitamins A, D, E, and K may be required. Therapeutic amounts of folic acid and/or B_{12} are needed in specific deficiency states including pernicious anemia. Pathologic conditions of the intestines that require bowel resection or intestinal bypass will require vitamin therapy, the specific needs being dictated by the location of the bowel resection. In burn victims and patients with extensive wounds to heal, vitamin C along with the B vitamins are frequently prescribed.

Thus, a number of specific deficiency states do require vitamin therapy. To date, though, no conclusive evidence has been found to indicate that multivitamin preparations or megavitamin dosages have ever helped a patient. In fact, much critical research is immediately needed to be certain that no harmful effects are being sustained by such practices. The toxic effects of excessive intake of vitamins A, D, and folic acid are known and, thus, the Food and Drug Administration restricts the amounts of these vitamins available over the counter. The question remains unanswered, however, regarding the possible harmful effects of prolonged megavitamin doses of any of the other vitamins.

The Vitamin C Controversy

No vitamin has a more historical past or controversial present than vitamin C. This vitamin that occurs naturally in citrus fruits such as oranges, lemons, and limes was first recognized by James Lind, a physician in the eighteenth-century British Navy, who linked its deficiency with scurvy, the dreaded sailor's disease. During the era of the great sailing ships, sailors deprived of fresh fruit and vegetables for months on end developed scurvy, manifested by fatigue, easy bruising of the skin, and bleeding from the gums and mucous membranes. The scourge of the British Navy two hundred years ago, this disease was greatly relieved by discovery that fresh fruit such as limes would prevent it. The British sailors' use of limes earned them the nickname "Limeys." Although the protective value of limes was discovered in the 1700s, the specific protective agent in the lime was not identified as vitamin C until 1932.

Today, vitamin C is in the news again as the Nobel Prize winning scientist Dr Linus Pauling has proclaimed that large doses of vitamin C aid the body's defense mechanisms against infection. Controversy rages, but no conclusive proof exists that vitamin C in megadoses protects against the common cold or any other infection.

While the average non-exercising person may not need to supplement his diet with vitamin C, it has been shown[6] that persons who engage in high levels of physical stress or consume large quantities of alcohol deplete the body's stores of vitamin C. Smoking and even chewing tobacco, if the tobacco juice is swallowed, also lower vitamin C levels. A diet high in charbroiled beef contains cholesterol oxide, a powerful oxidizer that quickly depletes both vitamins C and E. Our bodies cannot manufacture vitamin C; it must be ingested. Thus, it comes as no surprise that most athletes involved in endurance sports take supplemental vitamin C at the rate of 500 mg to 1 gm per day.

A recent poll of members of the American Medical Joggers Association preparing for the Boston Marathon revealed that over 90% of them took vitamin C as a supplement. While no scientific proof exists, still many trainers and endurance athletes feel that supplemental vitamin C greatly reduces the incidence of muscle and tendon injuries. Vitamin C has also been implicated in the pathogenesis of atherosclerosis. A deficiency of vitamin C may allow the lining of arteries (the endothelium) to degenerate and form sites for arteriosclerotic deposits.

From a medical standpoint, no harm is done since excesses of vitamin C the body cannot use are promptly excreted in the urine. Indeed, for the vigorously exercising individual, 500 mg to 1 gm of vitamin C per day may well be beneficial. However, I must caution that ingestion of more than 4 gm per day has been associated with kidney stones, thus massive amounts are distinctly discouraged.

CHOLESTEROL, HOMOCYSTEINE, VITAMIN B$_6$, AND ATHEROSCLEROSIS

Currently, one of the most hotly contested scientific debates involves the homocysteine theory and the role of vitamin B$_6$ in the prevention of atherosclerosis. Homocysteine, a very toxic substance, is regularly produced from methionine, one of the amino acids that constitute all of the protein that we eat. Since the body does not manufacture methionine, it must be obtained from dietary sources. Normally, homocysteine is quickly converted to cystathionine, a nontoxic substance used in other biochemical reactions. Vitamin B$_6$ acts as a coenzyme or facilitator of the enzyme reaction that converts homocysteine to cystathionine. A deficiency of vitamin B$_6$ leads to a reduction in conversion to cystathionine, a buildup of homocysteine in the blood, and the appearance of an oxidized form of homocysteine in the urine.

Kilmer McCully, a professor of pathology at Harvard Medical School, is generally credited with suggesting homocysteine is the cause of atherosclerosis. He proposed in 1969 that too little vitamin B$_6$ would retard the conversion of homocysteine to cystathionine, lead to a buildup of homocysteine in the blood, and thus promote atherosclerosis. Implicit in this theory were several predictions as well as explanations of findings.

1. If homocysteine is maintained in the blood of experimental animals, atherosclerosis should develop.

2. Humans and experimental animals eating diets deficient in vitamin B_6 should build up homocysteine in their blood.

3. People proven to have atherosclerosis, such as coronary patients, ought to show a tendency toward low vitamin B_6 in their blood.

In the last decade, each of these postulates has been found to be true, and thus the theory is gaining momentum. While a precise explanation of how homocysteine exerts its effects at the molecular level remains to be elucidated, the theory is alive and well, holding up nicely to its challenges.

Vitamin B_6 is plentiful in fruits and vegetables, less so in meats and dairy products. At a glance, it would seem unlikely that many people would be deficient in vitamin B_6. It must be realized, though, that 80% to 90% of vitamin B_6 is lost in milling wheat to white flour. Cooking vegetables inactivates two-thirds of their vitamin B_6, and cooking meat destroys 45% of the vitamin. Thus, it comes as no surprise that there are studies that show most Americans eating "normal" diets do not have adequate levels of vitamin B_6. This has been found to be especially the case in older Americans.

The homocysteine theory suggests most Americans eat too much protein and not enough vitamin B_6. It appears that a new criteria for selection of foods is on the horizon, not based just on cholesterol but on the relative B_6 and protein content (Table 4-2). While 2 mg/day of vitamin B_6 is currently an adequate daily amount, many Americans eat less than 2 mg/day and there is considerable evidence to suggest this level is too low to cover safely the entire adult population. Clearly, those groups prone to vitamin B_6 deficiency, ie, pregnant and nursing mothers, women on a contraceptive pill, dieters especially those on a high protein regimen, and old people, should receive more than 2 mg/day. Present evidence suggests that 10 mg/day of vitamin B_6 would provide a more appropriate margin of safety. Such a level would require a vitamin supplement, as it would not easily be found in our diet. Such levels are quite safe, as excessive vitamin B_6 is rapidly eliminated and the toxic dose of the vitamin is more than 1000 times greater than 10 mg/day.

Table 4-2
Vitamin B_6 and Methionine Content of Some Foods

Food	B*	M‡	B/M†	Standard portion
Apple	.03	4	7.5	150 gm
Avocado	.42	19	22	123 gm
Banana	.51	11	46	150 gm
Beans, raw snap	.08	28	2.9	125 gm; 1 cup
Beef, raw round	.50	970	0.5	85 gm; 3 oz
Bread, white	.04	126	0.3	23 gm; 1 slice
Bread, whole wheat	.18	161	1.1	23 gm; 1 slice
Broccoli, raw	.19	54	3.6	150 gm; 1 cup
Butter	.003	21	0.1	7 gm; 1 pat
Carrots	.15	10	15	50 gm
Cheese, cheddar	.07	653	0.1	17 gm; 1 in. cube
Chicken	.5	537	0.9	76 gm; ½ breast
Egg, hard-cooked	.11	392	0.3	50 gm
Lettuce, head	.07	4	17	220 gm; 4 in. head
Milk, cow whole	.042	83	0.5	244 gm; 1 cup
Oranges, raw	.06	2.7	22	210 gm; 3 in. dia
Peanut butter	.33	265	1.2	16 gm; 1 tbsp
Peas, raw	.18	44	4.1	160 gm; 1 cup
Potato, raw	.25	25	10	100 gm
Spinach, raw	.28	54	5.2	180 gm
Tomato, raw	.10	8	12.5	150 gm
Yogurt, plain	.032	102	0.3	246 gm; 1 cup

*Vitamin B_6 (mg/100 gm).
‡Methionine (mg/100 gm).
†Ratio of B_6 to methionine (× 1000).

A great deal remains to be learned about homocysteine. Conclusive proof of the theory awaits not only a molecular understanding of its action on the cells of blood vessels, but also conclusive results from large-scale clinical testing over a number of years. Still, with the cholesterol theory experiencing a renewed challenge and having inadequacies in explaining all aspects of atherosclerosis, the homocysteine theory deserves serious consideration. It is suggested that a lower intake of protein and a higher amount of vitamin B_6 may be desirable. Indeed, even in following a low-cholesterol diet, one would be helped, as a tendency toward lower protein intake will result.

Is the Cholesterol Theory in Trouble?

In a recent *New England Journal of Medicine article*,[7] Dr George Mann of Vanderbilt University Medical School wrote:

> A generation of research on the diet-heart question has ended in disarray. The official line since 1950 for management of the epidemic of coronary heart disease had been a dietary treatment. Foundations, scientists, and the media, both lay and scientific, have promoted low fat, low cholesterol polyunsaturated diets, and the epidemic continues unabated, cholesterolemia in the population is unchanged, the clinicians are unconvinced of efficacy....This litany of failures must lead the clinician to wonder where the proper research and solutions lie. The problem of coronary heart disease is real enough here, and yet it is rare in less developed societies. What aspect of life-style here makes atherosclerosis so malignant, its clinical consequences so fearsome?*

This highly controversial paper sparked an almost unprecedented flood of letters to the editor. Certainly, the cholesterol hypothesis still claims the majority of physicians as supporters, but many have retreated to a position where dietary cholesterol is only one of the more prominent of several risk factors in atherosclerosis.

*Reprinted, by permission, from *The New England Journal of Medicine* 291:178, 1974.

The cholesterol theory is traced back to a Russian I.A. Ignatovski who, in 1808, was the first to demonstrate experimentally in rabbits that a high protein, high fat, high cholesterol diet rapidly caused arteriosclerosis. His results were quickly confirmed, but his assumption that protein played a major role was never accepted. When Anitschkow and Chalatow in 1813 produced rapid arteriosclerosis in rabbits by feeding them high cholesterol diets alone, the basic model that high dietary cholesterol causes atherosclerosis was off and winging and has been popular ever since. It made no difference that others later showed feeding rabbits little or no cholesterol, but high protein diets even more rapidly produced atherosclerosis; the cholesterol theory remained in popular acceptance.

Why is the cholesterol theory being re-evaluated in 1980? The answer lies in the fact that several very large lengthy studies, one by the Mayo Clinic and the other the Framingham Study sponsored by the National Institutes of Health found little detectable relationship between diet cholesterol and serum cholesterol for people on a "normal" daily diet. This actually should not come as a great surprise, as cholesterol is not a foreign substance; most is synthesized by the body itself rather than derived from dietary sources. Our bodies will manufacture up to 1800 mg of cholesterol daily if none is eaten, and the amount our bodies produce drops as the amount we ingest increases. Thus, on a "normal" diet, it should come as no shock that one's cholesterol level may be higher or lower depending on other factors, ie, exercise, smoking, genetics, fiber in diet, and so forth. Even more important when considering atherosclerosis is that while a diet low in cholesterol or employing cholesterol-lowering products, such as fiber and yogurt, may result in a 10% to 15% reduction in serum cholesterol, is this really significant? The serum cholesterol levels in Americans are clearly 100% to 200% above the New Guinean highlanders in whom atherosclerosis is rare. Therefore, perhaps, no wonder the small 10% to 15% reduction in serum cholesterol associated with even the strictest diets does not seem to make a major impact on the rate of atherosclerosis.

DIETARY FIBER—IS TODAY'S DIET DEFICIENT?

The most significant food sources of fiber are unprocessed wheat bran, unrefined breakfast cereals, and whole wheat and rye flours. Additional sources include fresh and dried fruit, raw vegetables, and legumes. It appears that of all the sources, wheat bran is the most effective in increasing fecal bulk. This has led to commercial products of wheat bran on the grocery shelf with recommendations to add 6 teaspoons daily to everything from soup to chiffon cake.

Why is fiber important in our diet? Like many aspects of nutrition, there are known facts regarding fiber and other unproven speculations based on epidemiologic associations. First, let us review the hard data. Dietary fiber adds bulk to the diet. Because most sources are relatively low in calories, this means you feel full while you have consumed fewer calories than on a low-fiber diet. The increased bulk in your digestive tract greatly facilitates transit time. In one study[8] the transit time decreased from 48 hours to 12 hours when the same subjects switched from a low- to a high-fiber diet.

A high-fiber diet also produces stools that are soft, more bulky, more frequent (average of one bowel movement every nineteen hours), and contain twice as much carbohydrate, fat, and protein. This demonstration in man[8] that increases in dietary fiber or "roughage" increase fecal nutrient loss has been calculated to translate into energy losses that could account for an 8 to 10 lb weight difference over a one-year period. Thus, a diet high in fiber aids in weight control or reduction in two ways: it not only allows one to feel full with fewer calories consumed, but also affords a greater fecal loss of calories. There is a double reduction in caloric uptake by the body.

A high-fiber diet has been found to lower blood cholesterol and especially low-density lipoprotein cholesterol levels.[9] While some investigators suggest this is accomplished by impaired intestinal absorption of cholesterol and bile acids, reports are conflicting, and today it seems most reasonable to conclude that the mechanism by which dietary fiber lowers cholesterol is unknown. The fact that it occurs, however, raises speculation that the amount of fiber in the diet may be a factor in the prevention of atherosclerosis.

Unproven Provocative Theories
Regarding High-fiber Diets

The intake of crude fiber in the American diet has dropped 28% since the turn of the century.[10] While the intake of fiber from vegetables has remained relatively constant, that from potatoes, fruit, cereals, dry peas, and beans has declined. Coincident with this reduction of dietary fiber has been an increase in a host of ailments including coronary heart disease, cholesterol gallstones, diabetes, obesity, hiatal hernia, peptic ulcer, constipation, diverticulosis, hemorrhoids, varicose veins, and cancer of the colon. All of these have been linked to overconsumption of sucrose and highly milled starches and underconsumption of fibrous materials in the diet. While most of the postulates remain controversial and inconclusive and are based on epidemiologic relationships (that is, populations in the world with high-fiber diets who have a low incidence of these problems), it is still interesting to recapitulate the physiologic explanation.

Fiber, by adding bulk to the feces, will eliminate constipation and in over 70% of people render diverticulosis asymptomatic. To the extent the stool is soft and one does not have to strain, the problem of hemorrhoids is lessened. Obesity can be combatted by a high-fiber diet as previously discussed, and its control affords a reduction in adult-onset diabetes and problems of varicosities. The antiobesity and cholesterol-lowering effect of fiber are both cited to explain its beneficient effect on heart disease. The cholesterol-lowering effects account for the alleviation of cholesterol gallstones.

The transit time of feces may be a factor in hiatus hernia, ulcer, and most important colon cancer. In the last half century while the fiber consumption from fruits and vegetables has declined by 20%, and that from cereals and grains 50%, the incidence of colon cancer has risen significantly. Although unproven, much speculation exists that by decreasing the transit time through the colon threefold, the carcinogen or cancer-provoking agent, be it a virus or food breakdown product, is exposed to the large bowel for a much shorter period of time. It, therefore, has a diminished opportunity to break down the natural resistance of the colon and produce cancer.

Whether there is any benefit in preventing colon cancer or not, most Americans do need to increase the fiber content of their diets to achieve the known beneficial effects just discussed. While some may wish to sprinkle bran on various foods or substitute a fifth bran for an equal part of flour in any baked items from cakes to waffles, for most of us a significant increase in dietary fiber is achieved by enjoying unprocessed cereals, a slice of whole wheat bread, a nice salad, and some fresh or processed fruit on a regular basis.

DIETARY REQUIREMENTS FOR THE VIGOROUSLY EXERCISING ADULT

The basic dietary need for the athlete or vigorously exercising adult is increased caloric intake. This means larger servings of foods, particularly carbohydrates such as cereals, grains, and natural sugars as found in fresh fruit. Energy is provided less efficiently by fats, which should be mainly polyunsaturated, and least efficiently by protein. As indicated previously, the vitamin, mineral, and protein needs of most athletes are little different from sedentary spectators.

Water

Besides larger food requirements, the person who exercises strenuously also has an increased need for water. The amount depends upon air temperature and on the intensity and duration of exercise. While fluid should be replaced during vigorous exercise, it should be realized that the intestinal tract absorbs water at about 60 ml per hour. Thus, if perspiring freely, one cannot keep up with the water loss simply by drinking fluids. For this reason, endurance athletes such as marathon runners who know they will lose 4 to 8 lb of water during a given marathon, spend the hours immediately before the race drinking fluids until their urine is clear. They actually start the race with several extra pounds of water in their bodies that will quickly be lost as the race unfolds. Likewise, the vigorously exercising adult should precede his or her workout by drinking fluids. Remember that thirst is not immediately sensitive to serious body dehydration. Thus, plan your increased fluid consumption based upon anticipated fluid losses.

Roughly 60% of the adult's body weight is water. If daily weight fluctuates by more than 2 lb, then fluid has not been adequately replaced. Such a significant water deficit will compromise physical performance and even threaten physical well-being. Also, certain beverages containing caffeine (coffee, tea, cola, cocoa), as well as diets high in protein will increase urine production and even further deplete body water.

Salt Requirements

Too much has been made of the fact that we lose salt when we perspire. Actually, well-conditioned athletes lose only trace amounts of salt in their sweat. Habitual exercisers should not be concerned about salt needs so long as their diets are well rounded. Salt is ubiquitous in processed foods and already overly plentiful in most diets without ever reaching for the salt shaker. For most people, three daily meals easily replace the salt lost in up to 10 lb of exercise-induced sweat.

The Pre-exercise Meal

The pre-exercise meal serves the following needs: it minimizes hunger and weakness, ensures adequate hydration, provides for prompt emptying of the gastrointestinal tract, protects against stomach upset, and reflects individual food preferences. However, the traditional pre-game steak dinner is not recommended as a desirable nutritional preparation for vigorous exercise. The poorest source of energy, protein, compromises hydration by increasing urine, and the fat in meat delays emptying of the stomach and upper gastrointestinal tract promoting nausea and in some instances emesis.

Carbohydrates support best the glycogen and glucose stores needed for immediate energy and adequate blood sugar levels.

Carbohydrates rapidly empty from the stomach and do not produce urinary diuresis. Therefore, the best pre-exercise diet should include modest amounts of high carbohydrate foods taken at regular intervals with water or juices up to two and one-half hours before exercise. In the immediate two and one-half hours preceding vigorous exercise, it is best to consume no solid foods, but clear fluids may be consumed in limited amounts.

REFERENCES

1. Van Itallie, T.B., and Yang, M.U. Current concepts in nutrition diets and weight loss. *N Engl J Med.* 297:1158-1161, 1977.

2. DeWeese, V.A. No such thing as "localized" arteriosclerosis, say surgeons. *JAMA.* 238:571, 1977.

3. Yano, K., Rhoads, G.G., and Kagan, A. Coffee, alcohol, and risk of coronary heart disease among Japanese men living in Hawaii. *N Engl J Med.* 297:405-409, 1977.

4. Lieber, C.S. Pathogenesis and early diagnosis of alcoholic liver injury. *N Engl J Med.* 298:888-893, 1978.

5. Fletch, A.P. The effect of weight reduction upon the blood pressure of obese hypertensives. *Q J Med.* 23:331-345, 1954.

6. Kavanagh, T. *Heart Attack? Counter Attack!* Toronto: Van Nostrand Reinhold, 1976.

7. Mann, G.V. The influence of obesity on health. *N Engl J Med.* 291:178-185, 226-232, 1974.

8. Beyer, P.L., and Flynn, M.A. Effects of high- and low-fiber diets on human feces. *J Am Diet Assoc.* 72:271-276, 1978.

9. Munzo, J.M. Effects of some cereal brans and textured vegetable protein on plasma lipids. *Am J Clin Nutr.* 32:580-592, 1979.

10. Heller, H.P., and Hackler, L.R. Changes in the crude fiber content of the American Diet. *Am J Clin Nutr.* 31:1510-1514, 1978.

5   The Prevention of Musculotendinous Injuries in Runners

Lyle J. Micheli, MD

None of our panel has given more freely of his time than the next author, a former outstanding rugby player and now a prominent academic orthopedic surgeon noted both for his work in scoliosis and in sports medicine. Presently, he is the Director of the Sports Medicine Service of Harvard's Children's Medical Center in Boston. Recently, many of us watched him featured on a sports medicine episode of NOVA on Channel 2. Dr Micheli is currently the President of the New England Chapter of the American College of Sports Medicine and has just returned from being a visiting scholar at the University of Rhode Island. Dr Lyle Micheli will now teach us about the Prevention of Musculotendinous Injuries.

The growth of interest in fitness and exercise—in attaining it or maintaining it—is increasing throughout North America, as new and renewed athletes of all ages and both sexes run, roller skate, or "pump iron" as part of their fitness programs. While the majority have had some experience with athletics in the past, knowledge of training and conditioning techniques is often fragmentary or dated.

While specific sports preparation may be the goal of some of these athletes, most are interested in improving cardiovascular or endurance fitness, and avoiding injury in the process. A number of current sports, including cycling, swimming, cross-country skiing, and rope skipping can be used for cardiovascular fitness, and each has its advocates and proponents. But none of these approaches distance running or jogging in number of participants or relative convenience of participation.[1] This preponderance of runners and running is likely to persist for the foreseeable future.

Unfortunately, we are seeing far too many injuries from this presumably innocuous activity, ranging from bursitis and tendon inflammations to stress fractures and ruptured discs.[2,3] Further investigation has confirmed that body tissues are exposed to high levels of force—up to six to eight times body weight—with each footfall in running, and that these injuries result from the repetitive "microtrauma" of the foot striking the ground in runners who have trained inappropriately or have one or another additional predisposing factor such as muscle-tendon imbalance or pre-existing injury.[2,4]

In the more classic sports-related injuries—those resulting from single-impact macrotrauma—such as fractured collarbones, sprained ankles, or twisted knees, our traditional medical emphasis has been on the diagnosis and treatment of these injuries. More recently, studies of sports-related injuries, and of the overuse of microtrauma injuries in particular, have also attempted to determine, insofar as possible, the cause or causes of these injuries, as a first step in injury prevention.[5]

In our Sports Medicine Division at the Children's Hospital in Boston, we have developed a standard checklist of causal factors against which we compare every runner who presents with an over use injury. This checklist consists of six "risk" factors that may have contributed to the occurrence of a given injury in a given runner

1. Training errors, including abrupt changes in intensity, duration, or frequency of training.
2. Musculotendinous imbalance of strength, flexibility, or bulk.
3. Anatomic malalignment of the lower extremities, including differences in leg lengths, abnormalities of rotation of the hips, position of the kneecap, and bow legs, knock knees, or flat feet.

4. Footwear: improper fit, inadequate impact-absorbing material, excessive stiffness of the sole, and/or insufficient support of hindfoot.
5. Running surface: concrete pavement vs asphalt, vs running track, vs dirt or grass.
6. Associated disease state of the lower extremity, including arthritis, poor circulation, old fracture, or other injury.

This checklist has proven useful in both determining the probable cause of a given injury, and at the same time suggesting means of preventing the occurrence of other overuse injuries in the future. As an example, a runner with a significant leg length discrepancy may initially present with an inflammation of the anterior tibial tendon on the inner side of the foot and ankle of the short leg, and, if the discrepancy is not detected and remains uncorrected, may next be seen for an inflammatory bursitis of the opposite hip of the "long" leg.

When this checklist is applied to a given athlete presenting with an overuse injury, we have usually found that at least two, and sometimes three, of these risk factors are present. Although the novice athlete is more subject to overuse injury, any athlete at any level of performance or training may sustain an overuse injury. Thus, a nationally ranked distance runner who had decreased his level of training during a two-week exam period to 55 to 60 miles per week from a base of 90 miles per week sustained a tibial stress fracture when he immediately resumed his previous level of running. Additionally, he was found to have tight heelcords and hamstrings, admitted only to token stretching exercises, and had resumed running in a worn pair of racing flats left over from the spring track season.

THE MUSCLE-TENDON OVERUSE INJURIES

Muscles and tendons are truly inseparable. Every muscle is inserted into the bones that it moves by long (or sometimes short) fibrous attachments called tendons. Injuries of these muscle-tendon units can occur in the body of the muscle itself, at the junction of muscle and tendon, in the tendon itself, or at the site of tendon insertion in the bone (Figure 5-1).

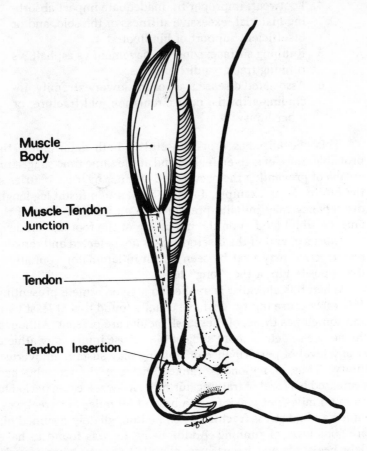

Muscle Body

Muscle-Tendon Junction

Tendon

Tendon Insertion

Figure 5-1 The muscle-tendon unit may be injured at any of four sites: the muscle body, the muscle-tendon junction, the tendon itself, or the site of insertion of tendon into bone.

If a muscle is exposed to excessive external stretch or excessive internal shortening of its own contractile elements, a muscle tear or strain can result.[4,6,7] While sometimes minimized by such terms as "muscle pull" or "charley horse," these injuries can be debilitating, and end a promising athletic season, or even a career. In runners, muscle strains often occur early in the season, and in runners who are tight and have not warmed up properly. In addition, runners who have not followed a balanced training program and have concentrated on strengthening one set of muscles without also strengthening the opposite ones are more likely to strain the weaker group. Sprinters and hurdlers, in particular, are subject to hamstring strains while the distance runner is more subject to quadriceps (thigh) and calf strains.

Tendons

In certain situations, the tendon may be the site of a chronic overuse injury. Usually, inflammation of the tendon, or tendinitis, is the direct result, although complete rupture of the tendon can occur. The pain and swelling of tendinitis is actually a normal healing process of the body in response to small tears or irritations in the substance of the tendon. Under normal circumstances, the pain and swelling are the body's way of obtaining rest for an injured extremity. Unfortunately, this pain feedback causes an inhibition of both the strength and flexibility of the muscle and tendon involved. Thus, a vicious cycle may begin in which the initial muscle or anatomic imbalance that helped cause the tendinitis is further exaggerated by the inhibitory effect of the pain.

In such a situation, the use of antiinflammatory drugs or, in particular, cortisone injections, must be approached with great caution. Though these agents may give temporary relief by decreasing the swelling or interrupting normal pain pathways, the primary condition usually persists. Unless specific training is done to improve the strength or flexibility of the injured muscles, more serious injury may result.[8]

A good example that illustrates some of these principles is that of Achilles tendinitis, or inflammation of the tendon of the heel. This condition occurs not infrequently in distance runners, and can be a very difficult condition to treat, once it has presented itself. This injury is often the result of a single episode of overuse, such as a workout with an increased mileage or rate of speed, or excessive hill work. This is an injury that must not be "run through." Proper initial treatment consists of relative rest of the muscle and tendon using ice compresses and mild anti-inflammatory medication such as aspirin. When the acute stages of injury have subsided, with a decrease in the swelling or pain, corrective measures such as stretching of the calf muscles and strengthening of the muscles in the front of the leg should be started. These improve the primary condition which is, at least in part, a muscle imbalance about the lower leg. In addition, attempts to compensate for anatomic malalignment, such as excessive bowing of the lower leg or excessive arch of the foot, can be done using specially made orthotic inserts that fit into the running shoe. If, instead of instituting these primary corrective measures, cortisone is injected into the tendon and no further corrective measures are taken, the medication may mask further small tears of the tendon, which can lead to complete rupture of the heelcord.[9]

Alternatively, repeated episodes of Achilles tendinitis, in which activity is resumed before complete healing has occurred and in which no attempt is made to correct the primary muscle-tendon or anatomic imbalance, can result in progressive scar formation to the point where surgery may be required to free up the tendon.

Muscle-tendon Avulsions

Complete or partial avulsion of tendon insertions from their bony attachments can occur in adolescent runners, particularly males. As a result of the second, or adolescent growth spurt, an increase in tightness or decreased flexibility can occur, particularly about the joints of the lower extremity.[10] This is due to the surge of bone growth at this time, and the inability of the muscle-tendon units spanning the joints to lengthen at a similar rate (Figure 5-2).

If one of these "newly" tight athletes participates in running—particularly sprinting or hurdling—without proper warmup or compensatory stretching exercises, complete avulsion of the tendon insertion may occur. The chronic version of this entity, which occurs at the site of quadriceps muscle insertion just below the knee, is called Osgood-Schlatter disease, and is frequently encountered in young male runners.[11]

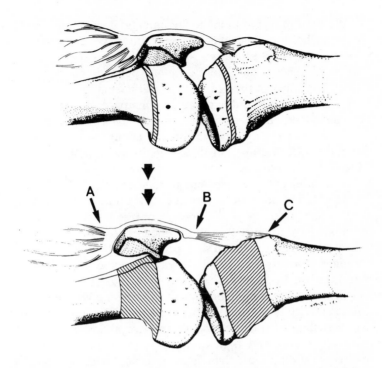

Figure 5-2 Overgrowth syndromes in adolescents. During the adolescent growth spurt an increased rate of bone growth from the growth plates, located at the ends of the long bones, may result in a relative decrease in flexibility across the joints, since the muscle-tendon units are secondarily put under tension by this growth. Pain and injury may occur at the insertion of the muscle into the kneecap (A), the patellar tendon (B), or the tibial tubercle, where the tendon inserts into bone (C).

PREVENTION OF INJURY

In running, as in many other sports, attention to four general principles of injury prevention is essential as a first step in reducing the rate or severity of injury. These include matching of participant to sport; specific training and conditioning; modification, if necessary, of running terrain or surface; and appropriate running equipment.

While running has much to recommend it as a simple and effective technique of aerobic fitness training, certain people are nonetheless constitutionally ill-matched for this sport. The current running boom has swept up many people who, because of limited flexibility in their hips, or foot abnormalities, are unable to run distances without experiencing many of the problems we have described above. In particular, we have found that people who lack inward and outward rotation about the hips have had difficulty with running. For these people, swimming or cycling, which does not require an inner and outer rotation of the hips, is a much better match of participant to sport.

As noted in our risk factors above, training error, including abrupt changes in intensity, duration, or frequency of training, is the single most important problem encountered in these running injuries. Proper attention to slow progressive training and conditioning is probably the best single way of preventing serious running injuries. In addition, supplemental muscle strengthening and flexibility training is important in someone whose primary fitness activity is running. Imbalances may develop in the runner consisting of relatively weak anterior abdominal muscles, relatively strong and tight quadriceps or thigh muscles, and relatively strong and tight calf muscles with a matching weakness of the muscles in the front of the leg and the back of the thigh, respectively. Supplemental exercises to increase the flexibility of the tightened muscles, and increase the strength and flexibility of the weakened muscles, is important in the general prevention of running injuries.

Little is now known about the impact qualities of different running surfaces, other than the frequent observation that excessive running on concrete pavement can be associated with the onset of overuse running injuries. Changing to asphalt or even dirt track or grass can often be instrumental in the resolution of pain and symptoms of these injuries. We often recommend a program of running on dirt or grass for the new runner, until the muscles, tendons, and bones of the lower extremities have been conditioned to impact with this more giving surface. Ultimately, road running on pavement can be performed with a relatively decreased risk of serious injury.

Finally, most of the recent studies on running injuries have served to emphasize that running shoes are not as important in injury prevention as some lay running magazines or shoe manufacturers might indicate. Training error and muscle-tendon imbalance appear to be much more frequently associated with this overuse injury. Properly designed running shoes, however, can be very useful in helping the body to compensate for some of the anatomic malalignments in the lower extremities, as well as to help in the impact absorption of the foot striking the ground. In addition, specially designed orthotic devices, which can be inserted between the shoe and the foot surface, can help to compensate for certain anatomic malalignments. These devices also increase the impact-absorbing qualitites of the shoe-orthotic combination, and are useful in helping prevent certain musculotendinous running injuries. Once again, however, these measures are well down the line as far as basic prevention of injury, and take a second place to proper intensity of training and frequency, as well as muscle-tendon training.

FIRST AID

It must be evident from the material above that despite appropriate technique and careful attention to their prevention, injuries can still occur. At this point, the initial care given to a runner can be crucial in reducing the extent of injury and the period of disability. The first few minutes may be the most important. Steps that can be taken to minimize further injury can be remembered by the initials ICE, which stand for immobilization, compression, and elevation. When taken together they also remind one of the need for ice application if available.

Immobilization, or rest, decreases the possibility of further injury to adjacent structures and can aid the mechanisms of the body that work to close off ruptured blood vessels and limit the extent of bleeding and subsequent swelling. A term that has been introduced into the field of sports medicine recently, "relative rest," implies a guarded and slowly progressive use of the injured structures while avoiding an intensity of use or training activity that can once again exacerbate the injury. An example of this might indeed be the recommendation that a runner who is suffering from an acute episode of Achilles tendinitis undertake distance swimming activities for a period of three to four times per week, during the first seven to ten days after injury.

Gentle compression dressings applied shortly after an overuse injury to a muscle-tendon unit can help to decrease bleeding and swelling. Dressings must never be so tightly applied as to obstruct blood flow or cause swelling below the injury. They can additionally assist in the immobilization of the extremity.

After a particularly severe injury, early elevation of the extremity can help to limit the initial injury and once again decrease swelling.

Finally, cooling of the injured extremity with ice packs or cold compresses also helps limit initial injury and swelling and provides pain relief. Intermittent cooling has proven most effective. Application of heat or other techniques such as ultrasound is generally reserved for a chronic injury and certainly has no place in the initial management of an acute musculotendinous injury in the first 48 to 72 hours after injury, as it may increase swelling by reopening blood vessels that were initially closed off following the acute injury.

REFERENCES

1. Buxbaum, R., and Micheli, L.J. *Sports for Life.* Boston: Beacon Press, 1979.

2. Brubaker, C.E., and James, S.L. Injuries to runners. *J Sports Med.* 2:189–197, 1974.

3. Guten, G. Herniated discs associated with running: a review of 10 cases. *Am J Sports Med.* 1980, (In press).

4. Turco, V.J. Injuries to the ankle and foot in athletes. *Orthop Clin North Am.* 8(3):669–682, 1977.

5. Micheli, L.J., Santopietro, F., Mariani, R., et al. Etiologic assessment of lower extremity stress fractures in sports. *Med Sci Sports.* 11:84, 1979.

6. Brewer, B.J. Injuries to the musculotendinous unit in sports. *Clin Orthop.* 23:32–38, 1962.

7. Burkett, L.H. Causative factors in hamstring strains. *Med Sci Sports.* 2:39–42, 1970.

8. Halpern, A.A., Horowitz, B.G., and Nagel, D.A. Tendon ruptures associated with corticosteroid therapy. *West J Med.* 127(5):378–382, 1977.

9. Jacobs, D., Martens, M., Van Audekercke, R., et al. Comparison of conservative and operative treatment of Achilles tendon ruptures. *Am J Sports Med.* 6(3):107–111, 1978.

10. Micheli, L.J. Sports injuries in the child and adolescent. Edited by R.H. Strauss. In *Sports Medicine and Physiology.* Philadelphia: W.B. Saunders, 1979.

11. Willner, P. Osgood-Schlatter's disease. Etiology and treatment. *Clin Orthop.* 62:178–184, 1969.

6 Economic Impact of Sports Injuries

Harriet G. Tolpin, PhD

It is with particular pleasure that I introduce the author of the next chapter, Dr Harriet Tolpin, the economist. She has recently contributed a chapter to the book Sports Injuries: The Unthwarted Epidemic *co-edited by Dr Vinger and Dr Hoerner, and published by PSG Publishing Company, Inc. Dr Tolpin will enlighten you on the Economic Impact of Sports Injuries.*

In 1978 the United States spent $192 billion on health care, approximately 9% of total expenditures in the economy that year. In 1978 almost 11 cents of every federal dollar expended went for health care. Since the mid-1960s the growth in health care outlays has in large part reflected substantial increases in health care prices; and for the past several years the rate of inflation in the health care sector has far exceeded inflation rates in other sectors of the economy. Concern over rising health care costs has intensified in recent years as both federal outlays and private health insurance premiums have risen along with health care prices. Whereas "access" and "equity" characterized the thrust of health care policy in the 1960s, "efficiency" and "cost containment" have become the focus of health policy in the 1970s and 1980s. With the shift in emphasis has come a serious reconsideration of the traditional focus of our health care system, a focus that has emphasized disease diagnosis and treatment. The conventional wisdom that "more and better health care services result in better health" is no longer accepted at face value. To quote from *The Surgeon General's Report on Health Promotion and Disease Prevention*, "...further improvements in the health of the American people can and will be achieved—not alone through increased medical care and greater health expenditures—but through a renewed national commitment to efforts designed to prevent disease and to promote health."

The relatively recent health policy emphasis on health promotion and disease and injury prevention has its origins in the hypothesis that, in economic terms, "an ounce of prevention may indeed be worth a pound of cure." The economist's perspective, which emphasizes the scarcity of resources relative to human wants and the necessity of allocating those scarce resources wisely, is being increasingly applied to questions of resource allocation within the health care sector itself. Might we not better allocate our limited resources toward health maintenance and prevention rather than toward disease diagnosis and cure? Prevention not only saves lives and improves the quality of life but can also save dollars (conserve resources) in the long run. To use the policymakers' jargon, prevention may indeed be the cost-effective strategy of maintaining and improving health status.

The focus of this book is health maintenance and sports injuries prevention. The benefits of maintaining health and preventing injuries may be viewed from several perspectives. For the individual, the benefits lie in avoiding the physical and mental consequences of illness and injury. Pain and suffering are, for the individual, primary costs, costs that can be avoided if such illnesses and injuries are prevented. It is not only the individual, however, and the individual's family, who incur costs from illness and injury and thus serve to benefit from prevention. To the extent that incidence and severity of illness and injury can be reduced, society also benefits. My task is to discuss the economic costs to society associated with sports injuries and thus to describe the potential economic benefits to society from sports injuries prevention.

Approximately 100 million Americans are involved in sports activities when both professional and amateur sports are considered. Estimates of the numbers of sports-related injuries are unreliable at best, and range considerably from more than 2 million to about 17 million. Estimates of the aggregate economic costs of sports injuries are nonexistent in large part because the data necessary to arrive at such estimates are unavailable. Calculations of the costs of sports-related injuries are, however, important primarily because many such injuries require a substantial amount of resources in their treatment and a significant number of these injuries can be prevented. Although protective equipment is widely available, the use of masks, helmets, and similar gear is often rebuffed by players and coaches because of inconvenience and the perceived stigma associated with such devices. Comprehensive cost analyses of injuries associated with particular sports can serve as an important aid in decisions relating to the allocation of resources directed toward the prevention of these injuries and can also provide additional arguments supporting the use of protective devices in sports.

ECONOMIC COSTS OF SPORTS INJURIES— SOME DEFINITIONS

An economist defines the "cost" of a good or service as the benefits foregone from other goods and services that cannot be produced because the resources have been used to produce the particular good in question. Thus "economic cost" is often termed "opportunity cost" in the sense that resources used in one way mean the sacrifice of those opportunities that would be available if resources were used another way. When the term "economic cost of sports injuries" is used, it refers to the opportunity cost that society incurs by diverting resources from alternative uses in order to diagnose and treat injuries associated with sports.

Economic costs of injuries are of two types: direct and indirect. Direct costs are those expenditures by the patient, the patient's family, and/or third-party reimbursement agencies for the resources necessary to diagnose and treat the injury under consideration. Direct costs of sports injuries thus include the costs of emergency room care, physicians' services, dentists' and other professional services, hospital care, drugs, medical supplies, physical therapy, rehabilitation services, and follow-up care.

Indirect costs are costs not directly associated with the treatment of a particular injury but rather those costs that are incurred as a result of the injury. These costs result primarily from reduced productivity and increased morbidity and/or mortality. The notion here is that there is a cost in terms of foregone output of those individuals suffering from premature death or disability as the result of a sports injury.

In addition to private direct and indirect costs, two other types of costs are relevant to cost-of-injury estimates: societal costs and social costs. Societal costs include insurance administration costs incurred by agencies and companies covering the incidence of selected medical events associated with injury, and legal and court costs associated with adverse side effects of treatment or product liability for injury.

The term "social costs" refers to psychosocial deteriorations that result from illness or injury. The concept of social cost recognizes, for example, that mortality influences the family and its life cycle, that morbidity may affect duration of marriages, and that significant associations exist among morbidity, economic dependence, and social isolation. Some injury victims may suffer loss of a body part, disfigurement, disability, impending death, pain, and depression. This person, as well as those around him or her, may be forced into a changed environment, economic dependence, social isolation, unwanted job changes, loss of career, and loss of education opportunities. Relocation of living quarters may also occur. Such changes are likely to induce anxiety and resentment, reduce self-esteem, and precipitate emotional problems. Mental illness may develop and family conflict and/or suicide may result. Disrupted development and delinquency may occur among children.

THE QUANTIFICATION OF ECONOMIC COSTS

In order to quantify the economic costs of a particular sports injury, it is necessary to first identify the injured person's diagnosis and treatment needs as well as postdischarge status. Figure 6-1 illustrates some of the possible variations in the course of diagnosis and treatment as well as in the residual impairment status; it also delineates resource needs corresponding to each phase of the patient's diagnosis and treatment.

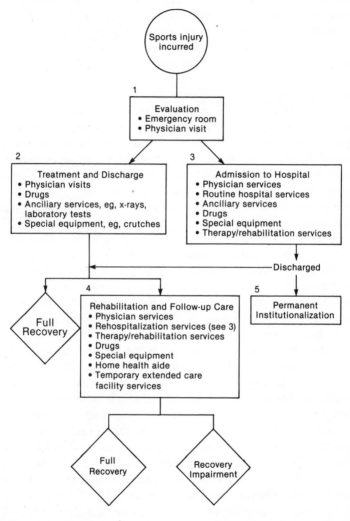

Figure 6-1 Treatment resource requirements of a sports-injury patient.

In order to identify the precise number and types of resources required (for example, the number of physician visits, the dosage and duration of specific drugs), expert medical opinion must be relied upon. The part of the body affected, the severity of the injury, and the age and physical status of the injured individual would all be considered in detailing the resource requirements for each type of sports injury.

In order to move from the identification of the direct cost categories to their quantification, estimates of unit costs of health care goods and services must be multiplied by the number of goods and services required.

Although indirect costs include several components, only a few items can be quantified. Morbidity and mortality costs are typically the largest component of indirect costs and are commonly measured in terms of the value of foregone output that sports injury patients would have produced if they had not incurred their sports injuries. Again, medical judgment as to the level of postdischarge disability and life expectancy is necessary in this phase of valuation.

Although the enumeration of societal costs may be conceptually straightforward, because of significant data limitations these costs are either not included in cost-of-injury estimates or are assumed to be some fixed proportion of expenditures in another direct cost category. To the extent that societal estimates are omitted, total economic costs will be underestimated.

It is in the area of quantification of social costs that much current methodologic discussion is being focused for it is in this area that the state of the art is least developed. Although some promising first steps have been taken in quantifying quality-of-life considerations through functional status indexes, and in inferring the intensity and duration of pain and suffering from assessments of the potency of required pain-killing drugs, relatively little has yet been done in terms of developing indicators of psychosocial distress and carefully enumerating the consequences of such distress. Psychiatric care costs and related costs of psychotherapy are, at this point, all that are available.

In order to compute the economic cost of a single sports injury, it is necessary to combine the available estimates of all of the above costs. In order to avoid the overvaluation of costs occurring in future years, economic costs extending over a period of years must be converted to a present value calculation by using an appropriate discount rate. While there is widespread agreement on the necessity of discounting future costs, there is no such agreement on which discount rate should be used. In order to compute the economic cost incurred by all patients sustaining a particular type of sports injury, estimates of incidence of sports-related injuries must be obtained and multiplied by the economic cost associated with each type of sports injury. Finally, in order to compute the total economic cost of sports injuries, incidence estimates and economic cost estimates for each sport must be aggregated over all sports.

In order to illustrate the use of the above methodology for cost-of-injury calculations, an example of how one would go about calculating the economic costs of a single sports injury is presented next. To provide continuity with the next chapter, the example chosen is that of an eye injury associated with ice hockey.

The Economic Cost of an Ice Hockey Injury—
An Illustrative Example

A 25-year-old man was injured playing ice hockey. He was hit in the eye with a stick. The injury ultimately necessitated a corneal transplant after which the player's vision was fully restored and recovery was complete.

The necessary steps in the evaluation and treatment of this injury were identified to include the following:*

1. Immediately following the injury the player went directly to a hospital emergency room where the injury was diagnosed as a severe corneal abrasion. The eye was patched and the patient was told to see an ophthalmologist the next day.

2. The patient saw the ophthalmologist, was given a complete eye examination, and told to return for follow-up.

3. In ensuing weeks the severe abrasion turned into a recurrent erosion and four further follow-up visits were required.

---

*Resource requirements were obtained from Paul Vinger, MD.

4. On the fourth follow-up visit, a soft "bandage" contact lens was prescribed.

5. Three additional follow-up visits ensued. The erosion treatment was not effective and the patient developed a corneal ulcer.

6. The patient was hospitalized for six days of intravenous treatment for the ulcer.

7. Following discharge the patient was seen another four times by the ophthalmologist for follow-up observation and further treatment.

8. The ulcer healed with a dense scar, significantly impairing the patient's vision. The patient elected to undergo a corneal transplant requiring five days of hospitalization.

9. The transplant was successful and treatment ended after four additional follow-up visits after hospital discharge.

In order to calculate the direct costs associated with the particular sequence of events described above, the resources utilized in each of the treatment steps must be identified and valued. This information appears in Table 6-1.

This example estimates the total cost of an injury that leaves no permanent disability, has a relatively short course of treatment, and does not result in significant morbidity. Thus the direct costs associated with the injury comprise the bulk of the total injury costs, indirect costs are relatively small, and no costs are incurred beyond the year in which the injury was sustained. In contrast, consider another type of sports injury, a spinal cord injury sustained while playing football, an injury that does result in permanent disability, significant morbidity, and costs, both direct and indirect, which are incurred over the lifetime of the injured player. For this injury both direct and indirect costs are substantial and recurring. The cost of such an injury may easily exceed $500,000.

AGGREGATE ECONOMIC COST OF SPORTS INJURIES— METHODOLOGY AND DATA REQUIREMENTS

Thus far the basic principles of cost-of-injury calculations in the case of a single sports injury incurred by one individual have been illustrated. In order to estimate the aggregate economic cost of sports injuries to the nation for a given year, it is necessary to 1) estimate the economic cost of injury associated with a given sport for all individuals injured while engaged in that sport for the given year, and 2) aggregate these cost estimates across all sports. The

Table 6-1
Economic Cost of an Ice Hockey Injury:
Severe Corneal Abrasion in a 25-year-old Man

Direct Costs*

Emergency room visit	$ 25
Complete exam by ophthalmologist	36
Four follow-up visits at $21	84
"Soft bandage" contact lens	180
Three follow-up visits at $21	63
Six days' hospitalization at $262 per day	1572
MD cost	156
Four follow-up visits at $21	84
Corneal transplant	
Five days' hospitalization at $262 per day	1310
Surgical fees	1248
Assistant fee	250
Anesthetist fee	260
Four follow-up visits at $21	84
Total direct costs	$5352

Indirect Costs

Work days lost at $68.30 per day†	
MD visits, 15 visits at ½ day each	513
Corneal ulcer treatment, 10 days	683
Corneal transplant, 21 days	1435
Insurance administration costs‡	210
Total indirect costs	$2841

Total Economic Costs $8193

*These costs are based on actual unit costs inflated to fiscal year 1980. Detailed calculations are available from the author upon request.
†Earnings data are based on Arthur D. Little, Inc. estimates prepared for the National Center for Health Services Research, Office of the Assistant Secretary for Health Research, Statistics, and Technology, Public Health Service, U.S. Department of Health, Education and Welfare pursuant to Contract No. 233-78-3013.
‡Insurance administration costs are assumed to be equivalent to 3.9% of total direct cost expenditures.

second task, that of aggregating costs across sports, is straight forward. The prior task, however, that of estimating the cost of injuries associated with a given sport, cannot be completed at the present time because of unavailability of necessary data.

In order to estimate direct and indirect costs of all injuries associated with a given sport, the first piece of essential information is an estimate of the number of injuries associated with participation in a given sport incurred in a given year. These injury incidence figures must then be classified according to age and sex of the injured persons, the type of injury incurred, and the severity of the injury. These classifications are germane because both direct and indirect costs for a given injury will vary by age and sex, and costs for different injuries will vary by type and severity of injury.

The second type of information necessary in estimating direct costs is resource requirements associated with the treatment of an injury of given type and severity for an individual of a particular sex and age. These resource requirements are then multiplied by per unit costs in the calculation of direct costs associated with those injuries. Where such direct costs are recurring, that is, certain treatment expenditures must be made beyond the year in which the injury occurs, these direct costs, appropriately discounted, must be multiplied by survival probabilities. For example, direct costs to be incurred two years from date of injury must be multiplied by the probability that the injured individual will be alive two years after the injury occurs. Survival probabilities in turn depend on the age and sex of the person injured, the type of injury, and its severity.

In order to estimate indirect costs, estimates of morbidity and mortality for the injured population are required. The most common way of converting these estimates into indirect cost figures is to use expected lifetime earnings tables that are available by sex and age groups.

To summarize, in order to calculate the direct and indirect costs of injuries associated with a given sport incurred in a particular time period, the following information is required:

1. Incidence of injury by age and sex,
2. Type of injury incurred,

3. Severity of injury,
4. Resources required in the diagnosis and treatment of the injury and per unit costs of such resources,
5. Morbidity and mortality estimates associated with each type of injury.

The above list of informational requirements points out the necessity for a consistent, reliable sports injury reporting system as a prerequisite to estimating the economic costs of sports injuries.

For sports-related injuries, data problems are particularly serious because consistent and reliable incidence data are not available. In conjunction with an injury reporting system, a mechanism for gathering information regarding health care resource utilization associated with the treatment of injuries also needs to be developed. One possible mechanism for doing this might be to record resource utilization data for selected samples of injured persons.

THE "VALUE" OF PROTECTIVE EQUIPMENT— AN APPLICATION OF COST-OF-INJURY ANALYSIS

Suppose we consider, in the context developed thus far, the "value" of the use of a protective device. In general, the benefits to be gained from use of a protective device are the costs averted because the injury does not occur. In valuing the use of hockey masks, for example, it is necessary to know 1) the costs of injuries incurred in the absence of hockey masks, and 2) the effectiveness of the masks in preventing or reducing the seriousness of those injuries. In order to estimate the benefits from the use of such a protective device, then, it is first necessary to compute the expected costs of the injury in the absence of the protective device. That is, the calculation of economic costs of specific sports injuries is a vital input for determining the benefits of a program or device or rule-change designed to eliminate or reduce the incidence and/or severity of those injuries.

At this point, it may be useful to consider a specific example relating to ocular injuries in hockey and hockey face protectors.

Paul F. Vinger, MD made a study of fairly typical ocular injuries suffered by 38 hockey players during a three-year period. For this group of injured players, the estimated initial direct costs involved in their treatment were, on average, $1586 per injured person. Assuming that 4% of all hockey players incur such injuries, the expected direct benefit from the use of hockey masks can be valued at $63.44 (.04 × $1586). When we compare this potential saving ($63.44) with the cost of a hockey mask ($20), we see that it is cost-beneficial to use the protective device. If, in this calculation, estimates of indirect, societal, and social costs averted through the use of such protective devices had been included, the benefit/cost ratio would be even greater. In general, the ratio of benefits to costs will be higher in cases where the cost of the protective device is relatively small and the effectiveness of the device in terms of preventing expensive injuries is relatively large.

THE NECESSITY OF A RELIABLE DATA SYSTEM

As is illustrated by the discussion thus far, the implementation of the economic cost-of-injury methodology is dependent upon substantial data requirements. Although a variety of systems do exist for the gathering and reporting of information related to sports injuries, none of these data collection systems was designed to provide national data representative of total injuries associated with a particular sport. Data that do exist either represent injuries associated with organized sports or injuries associated with unsupervised, unorganized sports activities. Much of the data that are collected, having been collected for specific purposes, are not collected in a form amenable to the categorizations necessary for calculations of economic costs.

Although clinical literature contains a wealth of information concerning the nature of sports injuries and available treatment regimens, relatively little data are available concerning the corresponding health care resources required in the treatment process, the costs of these resources, and the duration and degree of disability associated with the injuries. Such information is necessary for the calculation of direct and indirect costs associated with specific types of sports injuries.

Current research in the area of cost-of-injury appears to be directed toward the following areas: quantification of patient suffering in particular and social costs in general, valuation of different qualities of life, and development of more comprehensive and consistent data bases. The methodology of this type of analysis is fairly well developed to date; the binding constraint in the application of this methodology to sports injuries is the lack of reliable and consistent data. Those involved in the treatment and/or prevention of sports injuries must develop and maintain a reliable data system so that economic costs of sports injuries can be estimated and the economic benefits of protective devices can be ascertained.

SUGGESTED READINGS

Berry, R. *The Economic Cost of Alcohol Abuse and Alcoholism, 1971.* Contract HSM 42-73-114 (NIA). Rockville, Md: National Institute of Alcohol Abuse and Alcoholism, 1974.

Cooper, B.S., and Rice, D.P. The economic cost of illness revisited. *Social Security Bull.* Washington, DC: US Department of Health, Education and Welfare, February 1976.

Mishan, E. Evaluation of life and limb. *J Political Economics.* 79:687–705, 1971.

Mushkin, S. Health as an investment. *J Political Economics.* 70(suppl 5, part 2):129–157, 1962.

Mushkin, S.J., and Dunlop, D.W. (Eds). *Health: What Is it Worth? Measures of Health Benefits.* New York: Pergamon Press, 1979.

Powell, J. Pros and cons of data-gathering mechanisms. Edited by P.F. Vinger and E.F. Hoerner. In *Sports Injuries: The Unthwarted Epidemic.* Littleton, Mass: PSG Publishing, 1980.

Prest, A.P., and Turvey, R. Cost benefit analysis: a survey. *Economic J.* December:683–735, 1965.

Public Health Service. *Healthy People: The Surgeon General's Report on Health Promotion and Disease Prevention.* Washington, DC: US Government Printing Office, 1979.

Rice, D.P. *Estimating the Cost of Illness.* Health Series No. 6. DHEW. Washington, DC: US Government Printing Office, May 1966.

Schoenbaum, S., McNeil, B., and Kavet, J. The swine-influenza decision. *N Engl J Med.* 295:759–765, 1976.

Smart, C.N., and Sanders, C.R. *The Costs of Motor Vehicle Related Spinal Cord Injuries.* Washington, DC: Insurance Institute for Highway Safety, 1976.

Tolpin, H., and Bentkover, J. The economic costs of sports injuries. Edited by P.F. Vinger and E.F. Hoerner. In *Sports Injuries: The Unthwarted Epidemic.* Littleton, Mass: PSG Publishing, 1980.

Vinger P.F. Ocular injuries in hockey. *Arch Ophthalmol.* 94:74–76, 1976.

Zeckhauser, R. Procedures for valuing lives. *Public Policy.* 23:419–464, 1975.

7 Prevention of Eye and Face Injuries

Paul Vinger, MD

The next author is a longtime personal friend whose multiple contributions to ophthalmology, sports medicine, education, and the Emerson Hospital scene I have long admired. He has recently co-edited a book with Dr Hoerner and is responsible for all the mandatory face masks in youth amateur hockey. He was recently voted as the 1979 Massachusetts Ophthalmologist of the Year. Dr Paul Vinger, author, artist, activist will enlighten you on the Prevention of Face and Eye Injuries.

The attitude of many athletes is exemplified in my uncle Gus. Seventy-two-year-old Gustov, a former blacksmith from East Prussia, would demonstrate his tremendous strength by lifting the back ends of cars. A superior athlete in his own way, Gustov would stand a little taller when he rubbed his index finger over the diagonal scar that went across his cheek and his upper lip. How I used to listen to him in awe and amazement when he told me how he was cut while dueling in East Prussia.

Gustov's scar is a monument to the prowess of youth, a reminder of his old blacksmith days as the town tough and swordsman. He smiled with scorn when he told me how the other kids made phony scars with a razor. Gustov's perfectly placed scar is a source of tremendous pride. Who would dare suggest that one be deprived of such pleasure? To this day I would risk ridicule if I went to Uncle Gustov and even hinted that he could have avoided the injury. What if the sword had cut his eye? He would not hear any of it because the injury and the resulting scar are truly an essential part of his life.

Unfortunately, in some circles my Uncle Gustov's attitude still exists because sports injuries, especially those plainly visible, are worn like a badge of honor. The wrestler's cauliflower ear, the football player's gimp, the boxer's deformed nose, and the hockey player's toothless grin have a role to play in our American model of manliness. So, what does this have to do with the prevention of eye injuries in sports? Until we change this basic attitude of American manliness protective measures against traditional injuries will be resisted. Ten years' experience has proven over and over to me that data, no matter how convincing, will fall on resistive ears as long as Gustov's attitude persists.

Yet, on the other hand, there are many parents, athletes, and coaches who believe, as I do, that sports for youth should be as safe as possible while retaining the fun, appeal, and excitement inherent in the game. It is to these people who can view data objectively that I present a brief overview of eye and face protection.

Can we show that eye and face injuries in sports really are a problem? Even though there is a major problem in studying sports injuries—gathering accurate, fast, reliable data—enough is available to make some conclusions. If we look at eye injuries, the National Society for the Prevention of Blindness estimates 112,000 school-aged children suffered eye injuries from sports in 1978. The National Electronic Injuries Surveillance System (NEISS) estimated (Table 7-1) about one-quarter that number because it polls emergency rooms and does not get data on injuries seen in physicians' offices. If the NEISS data are multiplied by four, one would see a truer incidence of eye injuries in this country, and if multiplied by 10 the occurrence of facial injury would be approximated.

The average sports eye injury costs well over $500, thus we are dealing with an enormous social cost aside from pain and suffering.

Racquetball, volleyball, and soccer have had a rapid increase in eye injuries over the past six years. Hockey realized a reduction in eye injuries because of face protection.

Table 7-1
Estimated Number of Product-related Eye Injuries Treated in Hospital Emergency Rooms for Selected Sports: United States, 1973–1978

Sport	Total 1973–1978	1973	1974	1975	1976	1977	1978
Total	126,268	16,743	17,417	18,047	22,385	25,268	26,408
Baseball	36,419	5288	5416	4755	5371	6918	8671
Basketball	19,869	2127	3370	2563	4037	3466	4306
Tennis, badminton, squash, racquetball	18,049	1679	1719	2751	3519	4699	3682
Football	11,961	1620	2018	1439	2275	2291	2318
Bicycling	7856	1069	1244	1783	923	1138	1699
Sportsball, not specified	11,382	1293	730	1318	3297	3137	1607
Gas, air, spring-operated guns	8081	1267	1552	1489	1288	1150	1335
Hockey, all kinds	6717	1832	1037	1251	651	629	1317
Volleyball	3028	332	34	315	438	1095	814
Soccer	2906	236	297	383	586	745	659

Note: From this table the following can be seen:
1. Hockey injuries are decreasing as a result of protective face masks.
2. Although hockey injuries have decreased dramatically to players wearing face protection, a significant injury problem remains for unprotected players.
3. An upward trend of injuries in baseball, basketball, and football.
4. A steady stream of injuries from airguns and cycling.
5. A steady increase in sports-related eye injuries.

Source: Unpublished data from the Consumer Product Safety Commission provided to the Operational Research Department, National Society to Prevent Blindness, New York.

Fortunately by the application of two very simple and basic principles, we can prevent 90% of all eye and face injuries. The first principle applies to sports where people are colliding with each other or riding in a vehicle and crashing, generating tremendous forces. Since the forces in collision sports exceed the ability of the face to absorb the energy, the only way to protect the eyes, face, and teeth in a collision-type sport such as hockey, football, or lacrosse, is to have the forces transmitted through a face mask into a helmet with a suitable suspension system. However, once the forces are transmitted to a helmet, the total package of head protection must be analyzed as to how the impact relates to the brain and the neck. For collision sports, the concept of *total head protection,* not isolated protection to the eye and face, must be pursued.

In the second group of sports, which have injury potential from fingers, elbows, balls, racquets, etc striking the eye, the basic principle of protection is preventing the eye from getting hit.

In the face are two structures that do not heal well when significantly injured—teeth and eyes. A lost tooth can be replaced with a fairly good prosthesis, but for a lost eye there is no functional replacement. Therefore, the main emphasis is on protecting the eyes.

Half of the eye (Figure 7-1) lies anterior to the orbital bone, so the eye must be protected from the side as well as the front. The first type of eye injury is a cut with a piece of something sharp such as the patient's own broken eyeglasses, therefore we recommend that athletes not use glass eyeglasses. Plastic eyeglass lenses tend to shatter less easily than glass.

A golf ball impacting on the eye (Figure 7-2) demonstrates a second basic mechanism of eye injury. The eye is hit with an object smaller than the orbital opening—a finger, golf ball, BB, the end of a racquet, and so forth. The eye suffers tremendous deformation and may rupture because the orbital force rises after the pressure within the eye. The worst prognosis of all is for an eye that has a large posterior rupture.

The third type of injury is caused by a blow from an object that is larger than the orbit. Some of this energy is absorbed by the bone and some by the eye (Figure 7-3). The figure depicts a tennis ball striking the eye, but it could be a fist, elbow, baseball, or softball, anything larger than 2 inches in diameter. It can be seen that the eye does deform from its normal position, but since the ball forms a seal at the bony rims, the orbital pressure is increased concomitantly with the pressure in the eye, and the orbital pressure helps to support the eye from rupturing. Frequently the thin bone below the eye will blow out. Tears in the retina are common since as the eye is compressed it is stretched sideways.

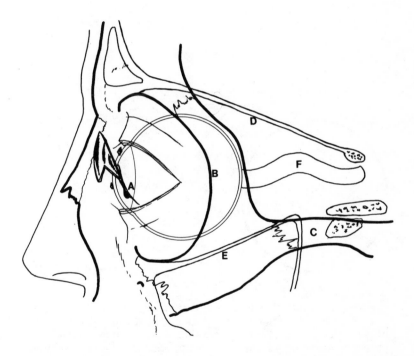

Figure 7-1   Direct blow to the eye (left eye, side view) by a sharp object (glass), with corneo-scleral laceration and iris prolapse (A). The drawing illustrates exposure of eye to injury from the side. The globe is relatively undeformed by the impact. (B) Lateral orbital rim, (C) zygomatic arch, (D) roof of orbit, (E) floor of orbit, (F) optic nerve.

FIRST AID AND EXAMINATION

To examine an eye that has a blunt injury, the physician must know precisely what the normal eye looks like and how to compare the injured eye against the mental concept of normal (Figure 7-4). This cannot be done by an emergency room physician; any blunt injury to the eye must be seen and followed by an ophthalmologist.

The basic principles of first aid for any eye injury are:

1. Look carefully.
2. Check the patient's vision.
3. Patch and refer.

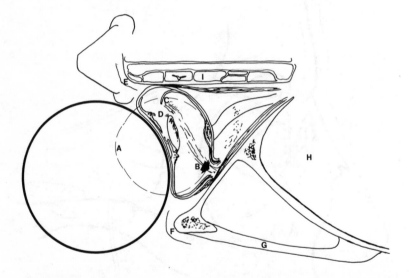

Figure 7-2 Direct blow to the eye (left eye viewed from the top) by a blunt object smaller than the orbital opening (golf ball). (A) Deformation of the globe by impact (normal position shown by dotted line). (B) Increase in diameter of the globe with release of greatly increased intraocular pressure by perforation. (C) Retinal tear caused by traction on vitreous base. (D) Rupture of lens suspensory ligaments. (E) Line drawn from medial orbital rim to lateral orbital rim (F) leaves about 35% to 50% of eye (A) unprotected by bone in blows from lateral side. (G) Zygomatic arch. (H) Temporal fossa (location of tip of temporal lobe of brain). (I) Ethmoid sinuses.

An example of the need for careful observation is the boy in Figure 7-5 who was poked in the eye with a finger. First glance shows what appears to be a lash on the cornea. A more careful look reveals the lens displaced from its normal position; the lash

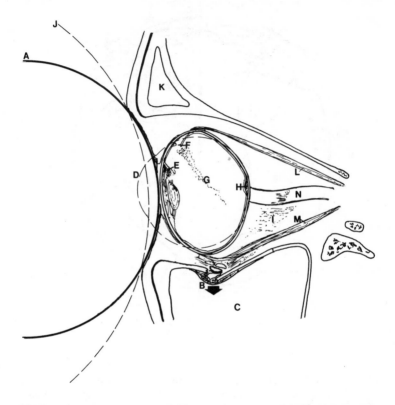

Figure 7-3 Direct blow to the eye (left eye viewed from side) by a blunt object larger than the orbital opening (tennis ball) (A). Ball forms seal at orbital margin, preventing release of orbital pressure except by fracture of floor of orbit (B) into (C) maxillary sinus; orbital fat trapped in fracture will result in diplopia. The normal position of the globe is deformed (D) with (E) resultant angle contusion deformity, (F) retinal tear, (G) vitreous hemorrhage, (H) submacular hemorrhage, and (I) orbital hemorrhage and edema. A ball larger than 4 inches in diameter (J) will not deform globe (D) as much, thus injury is less likely with objects larger than 4 inches in diameter. (K) Frontal sinus, (L) superior rectus muscle, (M) inferior rectus muscle, (N) optic nerve.

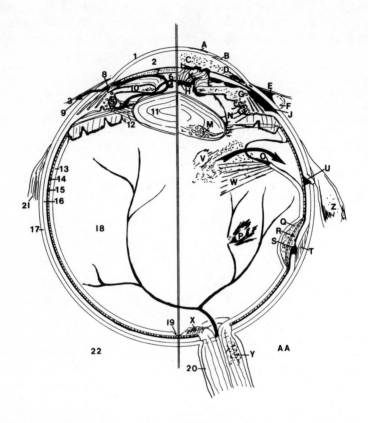

Figure 7-4 Left (numbers) is a normal eye, right (letters) is eye with typical injuries from sports accidents. 1. Cornea: (A) corneal abrasion, (B) corneal laceration. 2. Anterior chamber (filled with aqueous humor–plasma-like liquid): (C) cells and flare in anterior chamber (traumatic iritis), (D) blood in anterior chamber (hyphema). 3. Conjuctiva: (E) subconjunctival hemorrhage, (F) edema beneath conjunctiva (chemosis). 4. Normal aqueous circulation to nourish eye and maintain normal intraocular pressure. Ciliary body (5), through pupil (6) through trabecular meshwork (7) into canal of Schlemm (8) and out through conjunctival and episcleral veins (9): impediments to aqueous production and outflow (G) ciliary edema, (H) posterior synechiae (adhesions of iris to lens), (I) peripheral anterior synechiae (adhesions of iris to cornea), (J) angle contusion deformity and scarring of trabecular meshwork plus

blockage of meshwork with blood and inflammatory debris. 10. Iris: (K) rupture of iris sphincter, (L) iridodialysis. 11. Lens, and (12) lens suspensory ligaments: (M) cataract (opacity of lens), (N) rupture of suspensory ligaments with dislocation of lens. 13. Retina: (O) retinal tear with detachment, (P) retinal hemorrhages, (Q) subretinal hemorrhages or edema. 14. Retinal pigment epithelium: (R) subpigment epithelial bleeding or edema. 15. Bruch's membrane: (S) break in Bruch's membrane (choroid often also torn). 16. Choroid: (T) subchoroidal hemorrhages or edema. 17. Sclera: (U) scleral rupture with prolapse of choroid. 18. Vitreous: (V) vitreous hemorrhages and inflammation, (W) vitreous traction and fibrosis. 19. Macula: (X) Macula edema with loss of receptor cells. 20. Optic nerve: (Y) hemorrhage, contusion, or edema of optic nerve. 21. Extraocular muscle: (Z) hemorrhage, edema, or contusion of muscle. 22. Orbit: (AA) hemorrhage, edema, of inflammation of orbit.

---

is inside the eye; there is a hole in the iris; and the cornea is lacerated. If this athlete resumed play he could have expelled the contents of the eye through the laceration. Checking the vision, of course, indicated injury because the player could not see well with his lens out of position. With proper equipment the ophthalmologist could easily tell by making an optical cross section of the eye that the lash was, in fact, inside the eye and that the eye was cut (Figure 7-6). This eye, easily salvageable with sutures, could have been lost had the player returned to competition without very careful on-field evaluation. When looking at an injured eye one must really look. It cannot be a cursory glance.

The boy in Figure 7-7 who was hit in the eye with a hockey stick had a large hole in the retina. This injury demonstrates two important facts. First, his coach denied he was injured. The denial of sports injuries unfortunately exists because some people try to hide sports injuries for their own motives. Second, the line drawing shows the percentage of the retina seen by a physician who is not an ophthalmologist. He would totally miss the area of enormous pathology that requires special examination techniques and instruments.

To underline the point that all patients with blunt eye injuries must be seen by an ophthalmologist, a Canadian study of children with retinal detachment from eye injuries in sports

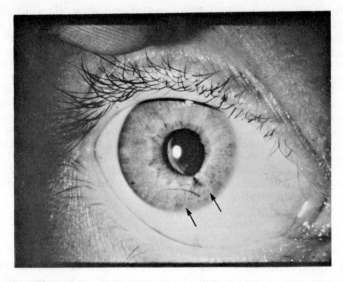

Figure 7-5 Subtile rupture of the globe. Note how the slit lamp enables easy observation of the lacerated cornea.

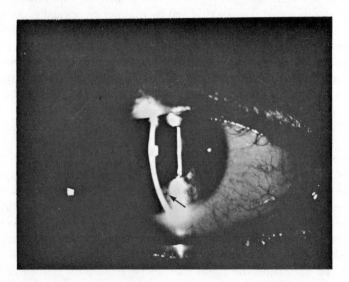

Figure 7-6 Same eye as in Figure 7-5. The lens is absent and the cilium (eye lash) is within the anterior chamber. All of these features would easily be overlooked on casual examination.

showed the average time between injury and diagnosis of retinal detachment was three years. By that time vision is often permanently lost.

PREVENTION OF INJURIES

Ice hockey is a sport with a high facial injury rate. Over 94% of professional hockey players have been hurt seriously in the face. The average professional player has had 15 facial lacerations requiring sutures, broken at least one bone in his face, and

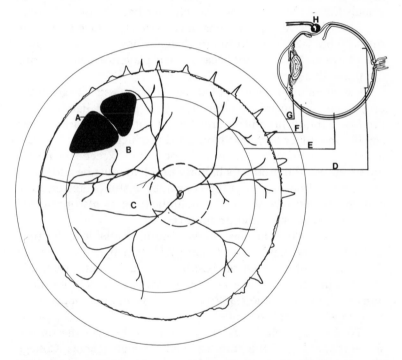

Figure 7-7 Drawing of retina of a player hit with a hockey stick. (A) Retinal hole, (B) detached retina, (C) attached retina, (D) area of retina usually seen by nonophthalmologist using direct (hand-held) ophthalmoscope, (E) equator of eye—absolute limit of view with direct ophthalmoscope, easily seen with indirect ophthalmoscope and condensing lens, (F) ora serrata, and (G) pars plana can only be seen by special techniques such as indirect ophthalmoscopy, and (H) scleral depression.

has lost two teeth. So, to play hockey without facial protection virtually ensures facial or eye injury. Many of these injuries can, however, be prevented.

Protection works—1.2 million hockey players wear full-face protectors in the United States and Canada; injury reduction to players wearing these items is over 99%; an estimated 70,000 injuries were prevented last year at a savings to society of over $10 million in medical bills. Appendix A lists manufacturers of good protective equipment. Most injuries to masked players occur with form-fitting goalie face masks. The form-fitting goalie mask is less safe than the wire face mask/helmet combination. Professionals know this but do not switch over because of tradition.

Many hockey organizations have mandatory face protection rules (Table 7-2). The old timers' leagues now have the highest risk of eye and face injury because their players are not wearing the protective devices.

Can all injuries be prevented? No. It is *impossible* to get 100% protection, yet an injury often triggers a product liability suit. Product liability premiums are driving out of the market some smaller manufacturers that have good products to offer but cannot stay in the business because the premium exceeds the potential profit. So, the product's liability problem must be addressed on a national basis so that the consumer is still protected from poor manufacturers while the manufacturer is also protected from exorbitant suits and premiums.

For hockey the cheapest, safest product available at this time is the fine-wire-mesh mask (Figure 7-8), which will not permit the entrance of a 2-inch blade, affixed to a helmet, preferably with a chin strap, that will not rotate. Available levels of protection are shown in Table 7-3. Protective devices must fit precisely to work at their full potential.

To decrease injuries further it is critical to get the professional model out of the grammar and the high schools. College players unfortunately are already professionals. But, in the high schools, grammar schools, and below the grammar school level, the pro model (win at all costs, play hurt, and use the best to win) should be discouraged. A substitute—have fun, play as safely as possible, and have everybody play—should be made.

The obligation to protect oneself does not rest only with the manufacturer or the health care professional; it must start with the intelligent person. I know a number of relatively well-informed, intelligent physicians who do not wear eye protectors

Table 7-2
Face Protection Rules of Various Organizations

Organization	Ages affected	Comments
Amateur Hockey Association, US (AHAUS)	6–18 (except 17–18 Junior-A Paid Gate)	Mandatory
Headmasters' or Principals' Associations (separate organization for each state in US)	14–19	Mandatory most states
Canadian Amateur Hockey Association (CAHA)	Same as AHAUS	Mandatory
National Collegiate Athletic Association (NCAA)	17–22	Optional
Canadian College Athletic Association	18–25	Optional
Eastern College Athletic Association (ECAC)*	17–22	Mandatory
Western College Athletic Association*	17–22	Optional
Central College Hockey Association*	17–22	Optional
Professional leagues	Over 18	Optional, used mostly after injury
Old timers' leagues, pick-up teams, etc	21–60 + children not in AHAUS or school game	Optional

*Would have to adhere to any mandatory ruling put into effect by the NCAA, which at the time of this writing is strongly considering mandatory facial protection for the 1980 season.

while playing racquet sports despite the fact that they have heard this all before. Many of us do not wear shoulder belts driving in our cars despite the fact that I can point out patients who have had low-speed collisions and lost both eyes hitting them on the steering wheel. We always think it will be the other guy that will be hurt, it can never happen to us—but it can.

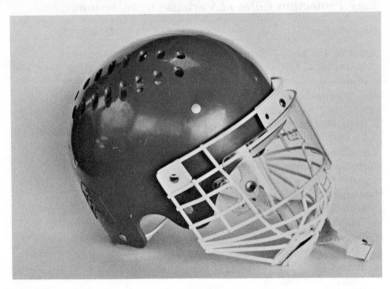

Figure 7-8   Full-face all-wire hockey protector.

Table 7-3
Levels of Protection

I. Collision sports
   Certified helmet plus:
   Safest:
   1. Hockey face mask, fine-mesh, certified HECC, CSA.
   Adequate:
   2. Hockey face mask, large-mesh, certified HECC.
   3. Football face mask.
II. Other sports:
   Safest:
   1. Polycarbonate industrial safety lenses (ANSI Z 87.1) mounted in industrial frame with clear side shields or polycarbonate injection moulded frame.
   2. CR 39 industrial safety lenses (ANSI Z 87.1) mounted in frames above (1).
   3. Plano injection moulded polycarbonate eye protector (Pro-Tec).
   Adequate:
   4. Polycarbonate industrial safety lenses (ANSI Z 87.1) mounted in industrial or sports frame without side shield.
   5. CR 39 industrial safety lenses (ANSI Z 87.1) in frames above (4). (Note: Industrial glass safety lenses are usually too heavy for athletes.)
   Adequate for tennis/badminton:
   6. Streetwear eyeglasses with plastic lenses.
   Not recommended for athletes:
   7. Streetwear eyeglasses with glass lenses. Pose definite hazard of eye laceration if struck with force.
   8. Contact lenses—offer no protection.
   9. Bare eyes.

SUGGESTED READINGS

Pashby, T.J. Eye injuries in Canadian hockey. Phase II. *Can Med Assoc J.* 117:671–678, 1977.

Pashby, T.J., Pashby, R.C., Chishom, L.D.J., et al. Eye injuries in Canadian hockey. *Can Med Assoc J.* 113:663–666, 674, 1975.

Vinger, P.F. A sporting chance with protective eyewear. *The Sight Saving Review.* 49(1):3–9, 1979.

Vinger, P.F., and Hoerner, E.F. (Eds.) *Sports Injuries: The Unthwarted Epidemic.* Littleton, Mass: PSG Publishing, 1980.

8 The Prevention and Treatment of Upper Extremity Athletic Injuries

Earl F. Hoerner, MD

Our next author is board-certified in multiple specialties and possesses a curriculum vitae so thick one requires bookends to contain it. Presently, he is Professor of Sports Medicine at Tufts University and Director of the Sports Medicine Clinic at Braintree Hospital in the metropolitan Boston area. His wisdom is sought by many and appreciated by all. He enjoys a reputation within the field of sports medicine by those who know him personally as the godfather because he is so giving of his time and his efforts. Professor Earl Hoerner will talk to you on the prevention and treatment of upper extremity injuries.

The art of throwing, fly casting, or using a racquet to hit a ball or similar object is an integral aspect of many popular sports and recreational activities. An example is the sport of baseball where throwing is considered a primary skill. Fifty percent of all injuries result from the throwing motion. The upper extremity mechanism acts in a synergetic action with other anatomic parts of the body in the final action to hit, throw, or propel a ball or other object with accuracy, speed, and distance. These actions of the entire body are complex, and to derive the final action of the upper extremity involves the sequencing and coordination of the entire body. As the sporting activity is performed, the various segments of the body act in varying degrees depending on the weight of the object to be thrown or the object to be hit by the racquet. In an activity such as the hammer throw, the body segments function in a different manner than in throwing a baseball, softball, or discus, casting a fly, or using a squash racquet.

The kinetic action of the upper extremity in performing these motions consists mainly of four steps, and occurs in a sequential manner. They are as shown in Figure 8-1.

1. Wind-up,
2. Cocking,
3. Acceleration,
4. Follow-through.

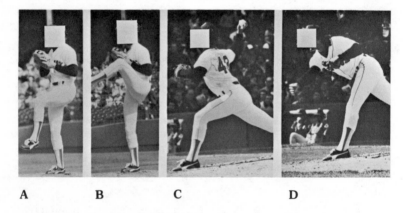

A   B   C   D

Figure 8-1 Demonstration of phases of **A** wind-up, **B** cocking, **C** acceleration, and **D** follow-through.

In Chapter 5 Dr Micheli discussed the lower extremities and soft tissue injuries and how one carries out biomechanical analysis of the prevention, diagnosis, and treatment of such injuries. His comments are also appropriate for musculotendinous and other similar upper extremity injuries. The principles of biomechanics hold for all segments of the body.

SHOULDER INJURIES

The shoulder is one of the most mobile joints in the body. It has a wide range of motion, in elevation, forward flexion, backward extension, internal and external rotation, and also adduction and abduction. The combination of these motions is termed circumduction. In the act of throwing the shoulder acts as a base for the arm to rotate about and functions, therefore, as a fulcrum. The final integrated action of throwing is a modified circumduction pattern. The rhythm through the phases is progressive and should be performed smoothly. This range and combination of motions, plus the repetitiveness of an athletic activity, is responsible for the wide range of injuries that occur in actions such as throwing or fly casting.

The source of power in the shoulder is the musculotendinous units, and the majority of injuries involve these soft tissue structures. Injuries to the muscles, tendons, ligaments, and capsule can occur when the tissue is stretched repetitively and fatigue occurs, or when the tissue becomes stretched beyond its limit of elasticity. Another mechanism that is unique to this anatomic area of the body occurs with impingement of the soft tissues between opposing bony structures such as the acromion and the rim of the glenoid. In the heavier throwing sports such as the hammer throw or discus, more extensive injuries may occur such as rotator cuff tears, subluxations, or dislocations. However, strains, sprains, tendinitis, and even myositis ossificans (Figure 8-2), are also common in all athletic activities involving the throwing motion.

Each injury of the shoulder girdle and upper arm must be analyzed and treated in an individual manner. Consideration and deliberation must be given to body type, ie, whether the patient is a hyperflexible, loose-jointed adolescent, or a middle-aged adult with degenerative joint disease and associated contractures of the soft tissues. In addition, age, state of fitness, physical conditioning, the playing environment, role of protective and playing equipment, and the anatomic structures must be reviewed, correlated, and integrated to properly understand the injury of the participant.

As an example, in order to understand and then classify shoulder injuries in softball, the shoulder must be separated into various but distinct anatomic units. These include the joints—scapulothoracic, acromioclavicular, glenohumeral, and sterno-clavicular. The soft tissues are separated into the musculotendinous and ligamentous structures. These soft tissues are also subdivided into anterior and posterior components. Injuries in this category are the common entities known as calcified supra-spinatous tendon, sub-deltoid bursitis, or tendinitis of the biceps or triceps muscle insertions.

Using this anatomic tissue classification, and considering the phase of the arm and shoulder motion in which the injury was sustained or pain occurred, definitive analysis can be performed. For example, in the early wind-up and cocking phases, few injuries are sustained. However, a local bursitis may occur at the superior medial border of the scapulae causing a scapulothoracic joint irritation. This can develop into what is commonly called the "snapping scapula syndrome."

While proceeding from the wind-up to the cocking phase, the posterior soft tissue structures contract, while the anterior

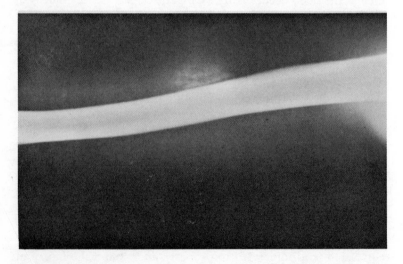

Figure 8-2 Myositis ossificans of upper arm in a high school hammer thrower.

structures relax, and subsequently the anterior structures are placed under stretch. All this happens while the humeral head of the upper arm is elevated into the glenoid socket. These synergistic muscle and bone actions must function in a coordinated manner, and any disruption such as seen in soft tissue contracture will cause extensive distress in the throwing mechanism. When excessive stretching or a loose joint occurs, subluxation either posterior or anterior may result. The subluxation may progress to a complete dislocation.

The anterosuperior structures that are potential candidates for injury are the anterior capsule and subscapular tendon, the glenohumeral ligament, the pectoralis major, the anterior deltoid, the latissimus dorsi, the teres major, and the long head of the biceps.

The pectoralis major, if overdeveloped as by excessive weight training, when contracted may tear at its insertion into the humerus, posterior to the biceps groove, or at its clavicular origin. Rarely the muscle belly itself may tear. During the early acceleration phase with violent contracture, the anterior deltoid muscle may be torn along with the pectoralis muscle. The subscapularis muscle and tendon unit also may be strained or torn as the acceleration phase is initiated and as this internal rotator muscle is maximally stretched and begins to contract violently.

The latissimus dorsi muscle, which is usually overdeveloped in the mature throwing athlete, has a tendency to develop a myostatic internal rotation contracture. This can lead to either a latissimus dorsi strain or tear. In the early acceleration phase of throwing, the biceps tendon may be forced to subluxate or pop medially on forced internal rotation. The tendon may subluxate out of the groove or after a time of chronic irritation, it may cause an osteophyte or bony spurring in the bicipital groove. This causes fraying of the tendon and a local irritation process in the biceps tendon.

It is probable that most shoulder injuries are brought on by overstretching in the cocking and early acceleration phases. In early acceleration, the humeral head may subluxate anteriorly, and as the acceleration continues, the impingement of the greater tuberosity under the rotator cuff structures beneath the acromion and the acromioclavicular joints may occur. Anterior subluxation or slipping of the humeral head occurs in immature or loose-jointed individuals that have a large wind-up and exert a powerful cocking and early acceleration force against an over-stretched arm. The humeral head is forced forward and actual subluxation can occur. This can be reproduced by examination. The humeral head can actually be lifted out of the glenoid cavity anteriorly in the motion pattern. Standard x-rays are usually normal and a definitive diagnosis depends on suspecting that the process is occurring. An arthrogram (Figure 8-3) of the shoulder, which is an x-ray dye study, and possibly arthroscopy, which is looking into the joint with the fiber optic instrument, may be necessary to demonstrate a stretching of the anterior capsule and a flattening of the back of the humeral head.

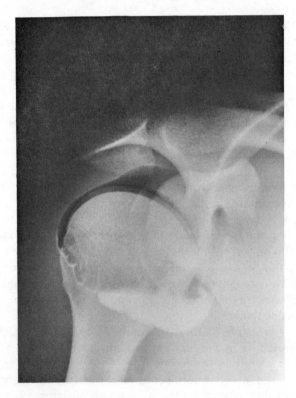

Figure 8-3 Arthrogram of shoulder.

With faulty motion or with uncontrolled motion acceleration, or with a long cross-body follow-through, the thrower can develop a chronic rotator cuff tendinitis. This is really an overuse syndrome due to an overloading of the rotator cuff tendons. Of importance is that this can lead to thickening and impingement of the tendon. When this syndrome develops, the first symptom noticed is lack of external rotation in the cocking phase. With the loss of external rotation, the athlete will not be able to get his arm rotated back as far as normal in cocking and, therefore, will develop a continued impingement throwing the ball with a short arc or range of motion. Fraying or partial thickness tears usually occur; rarely does there occur a complete tear of the rotator cuff.

Diagnosis is by positive physical signs of impingement by demonstration of cuff weakness, and demonstration of lack of external rotation in cocking. The arthrogram (Figure 8-3) is usually negative when fraying of the cuff is present, as the changes are not gross enough to show up. However, on arthroscopy there are findings such as a synovitis or irritation of the joint lining surrounding the cuff.

The structures that are involved in follow-through and release that can cause injury are the posterior cuff and capsule, triceps tendon, teres major, and acromioclavicular joint. Continual stretch and follow-through can cause stretching of the posterior capsule with resulting stretching of the capsule and posterior subluxation.

Minor repetitive tears of the teres major and posterior capsule can cause a painful calcification at the posterior glenoid. It may have to be surgically treated to get relief.

Triceps tendinitis can also be caused by forceful follow-through, or through an overuse syndrome. The acromioclavicular joint is also prone to compressive forces in follow-through. Continued trauma may lead to degenerative spurring of the clavicle with pain and enlargement of the joint.

There are two lesions seen less often but still worth mentioning, because of their seriousness. One is brachial plexus stretch. This can be seen in a pitcher, where after a certain pitch he will have a "dead arm." Examination may reveal multiple abnormal neurologic findings in the arm. The second is thrombosis of the subclavian or axillary vein. Additional tests (electromyogram or nerve conduction studies for nerve lesions, and venography for the venous lesions) are required for diagnosis.

ELBOW INJURIES

The elbow articulates with three bones, the humerus, ulna, and radius. It forms a hinge joint between the lower end of the humerus and the olecranon and coronoid processes of the ulna and head of the radius. This relationship between the two forearm bones forms a joint by which the radius can rotate around the ulna giving the motion of spination and pronation of the forearm. Joint stability and congruity are maintained by five ligaments.

Elbow injuries are most commonly connected with throwing mechanisms or direct trauma. Hyperextension injuries are quite common in both competitive and recreational activities. Repetitive throwing or racquet ball hitting may result in elbow joint changes in the bone, cartilage, fibrocartilage, ligament, or synovial membrane. Pitching effects can be classified into two main subsets: the adult, and adolescent or preadolescent.

As with the shoulder, the nature of kinetic stresses placed on the elbow can best be understood by a biomechanical analysis of elbow motion. To throw an object repetitively with control and speed requires coordination of body forces including the legs, trunk, shoulder, forearm, wrist, and hand. The four phases of wind-up, cocking, acceleration, and follow-through each have different forces. During the wind-up phase, the trunk is rotated away from the direction of the throw, and the body weight is loaded upon the opposite lower extremity. In cocking and acceleration, the legs are coiled in preparation for initiating the release. This is accomplished with an explosive rotation and thrust of the trunk in the direction of the throw. The shoulder, arm, forearm, and hand component assumes an abducted and extended attitude in relation to the trunk. During wind-up, significant stresses are not yet exerted on the upper extremity.

The cocking phase is characterized by transfer of body weight to the opposite lower extremity with thrust of the trunk in the direction of the throw. The throwing extremity lags behind, forcing the humerus into extreme abduction and external rotation. The elbow is flexed, thus enhancing the degree of torque and motion on the humeral shaft, glenohumeral shoulder capsule, and structures crossing the shoulder joint.

Owing to extreme external humeral rotation during this phase, extraordinary stresses are exerted on these structures. During the acceleration phase, the inertia of the trunk and legs is supplemented by contraction of intrinsic and extrinsic muscles of the shoulder. These combined forces whip the arm in the direction of the throw, with a violent force. During this phase, the biceps and triceps muscles as well as the forearm muscles support the stability of the elbow. However, this whip-like action tends to force the ulna and radius into an outward valgus attitude with respect to the distal humerus. This generates a compression force at the lateral radiohumeral articulation and a distracting force at the medial ulna-humeral articulation. This mechanism is responsible for medial elbow overload and lateral elbow compression. The repetition of motion can produce elbow injuries.

As the throwing motion progresses into the acceleration phase, compressive forces are exerted on the lateral aspect of the elbow joint at the radiohumeral articulation. The medial aspect of the joint is undergoing distraction forces attempting to open the joint space. As extension occurs, the movement and gliding of the ulna olecranon process into the humeral trochlear groove is one of valgus (outward) attitude. When performed repeatedly the normal relationship of the bone surfaces can finally disrupt and result in degenerative joint disease.

In the final phases of this upper extremity motion—release and follow-through—control and direction are applied to the ball or thrown object by the forearm and wrist action of pronation, and by flexion of the hand associated with ulnar or radial deviation of the wrist. The converse is true in hitting or using a racquet to hit a ball or object; extension at the wrist by the hand is the primary mechanism. These actions produce "tennis elbow" or lateral epiphysitis and "pitcher's elbow" or medial epiphysitis in the respective sports (Figure 8-4).

As mentioned previously, differentiation between preadolescent and adolescent elbow problems, and those of the adult, is based on the fact that growth and development complicates the picture in the former. In adolescence possibility of injury to the epiphyseal plate or growth center of the bone exists. This vulnerable link in the growing, maturing youth is quite sensitive to injury and should be considered the weakest link in the musculotendon-skeletal system. Therefore, trauma that can produce a sprain in an adult may result in a disturbance in the growth plate of maturing children. Repetitive forces acting over

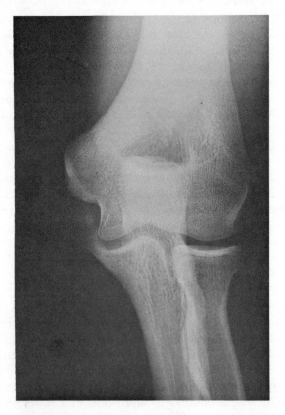

Figure 8-4 Elbow joint showing medial and lateral condyles of the humerus and humerus-ulna-radius articulations.

a long period of time may produce degenerative joint disorders in the adult and in a youth decrease the growth process and even facilitate premature closure of the growth plate.

Torg in his 1972 article published in *Pediatrics* classified "Little League elbows" into six distinct types. Three occur on the medial side of the elbow and result from distraction forces occurring during the acceleration phase of the throwing motion:

1. Growth acceleration,
2. Traction epiphysitis,
3. Avulsion fracture.

Growth acceleration reported by Adams in 1968 in *Clinical Orthopaedics* is considered to be a fragmentation of the medial epiphysis of the humerus. It occurs in a significant number of Little League baseball pitchers. An x-ray comparison of the non-pitching arm with the pitching arm of these youths shows a delayed epiphyseal closure of the pitching arm. The distraction forces of throwing the ball retard the growth center. Torg has drawn a comparison to the tibial tubercle epiphysitis of the knee known as Osgood-Schlatter disease.

The definitive pathologic finding seen in Little League pitchers is an avulsion fracture on the medial side of the elbow. This results from forceful contractions of the flexor muscle group (Figure 8-5).

Pathology may occur on the lateral side of the elbow joint because of the compression forces generated by the acceleration phase of the throwing motion. This may produce bony changes in the head of the radius or humeral condyle. It should be noted that these compression forces and resultant bony changes may also be seen in other youth sports such as gymnastics, wrestling, tennis, and racquet sports. The clinical findings are pain and swelling of the elbow and limitation of range of motion in extension or supination-pronation of the forearm. X-ray changes depend on the site and duration oɪ pathology. Torg in his detailed study documents that the pathologic changes that occur in the radial head are similar to those that occur in the hip joint in Perthes disorder, an avascular necrosis of the capital femoral epiphysis. First, there is a condensation and subsequently a sclerosis of the involved bone. This pathologic process progresses to fragmentation and radiolucency of the area, and finally deformity and resultant incongruity of the articular surfaces.

When diagnosed, treatment consists of immobilization for a period of time adequate to allow the radial head to regain vascular sufficiency and remodel the articular surface. If growth is complete, consideration may be given to excision of the radial head. The indications for surgery are loss of the congruency of the articular surface, and failure to respond to conservative care.

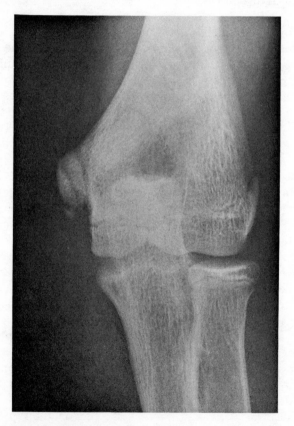

Figure 8-5 Avulsion fracture of the medial epicondyle at the origin of the flexor muscle group in a young baseball pitcher.

A second problem that may result from the compression forces on the lateral side of the elbow is osteochondritis of the humeral capitellum. The etiology appears to be the same as that producing radial head pathology. The athlete presents with symptoms of elbow pain and limitation of range of motion. The x-ray is diagnostic and reveals an area of radiolucency, and occasionally even the presence of loose bodies (Figure 8-6).

The third type of lateral elbow injury is "Little League elbow," the nonunion of a stress fracture through the olecranon

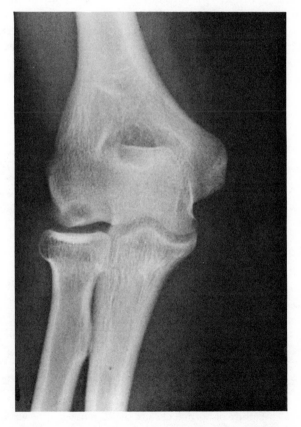

Figure 8-6 Osteochondrosis of the capitellum of the humerus in a young athlete.

growth plate. After the incurrence of a stress fracture as a result of continued lateral compression in the joint, a sclerosis occurs on both sides of the growth plate (Figure 8-7).

The forces that produce elbow lesions in the adolescent are essentially the same as in adults, but are of greater magnitude. Repetitive trauma over an extended period of time may produce degenerative joint changes, muscle strains, ligamentous sprains, and even myositis ossificans (see Figure 8-2).

Two additional problems are biceps and triceps tendinitis. Anterior capsular strain or biceps tendinitis is noticed, not only in the Little League player, but more commonly in the adult athlete. Strains develop over a period of time and are associated with an increase of the carrying angle, and a valgus deformity of the elbow. This is caused by lateral compression in the acceleration phase and develops in association with flexion contractures as a result of anterior capsule strain and/or biceps tendinitis.

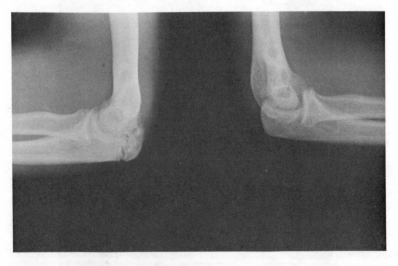

Figure 8-7 Failure of normal closure of olecranon epiphysis (left) with comparative view of a normal elbow (right).

INJURIES TO THE FOREARM, WRIST, AND HAND

Forearm injuries are usually fractures, strains, abrasions, or puncture wounds. A Colles fracture of the radius and ulna occurs from falling on the outstretched hand or using the hand to ward off another player. It requires the use of a cast for immobilization and as long as six to eight or more weeks to heal.

Most wrist injuries are either sprains or fractures. Differentiation is often only possible with x-rays and continued follow-up. Occult fractures do occur and even if the first x-ray is negative, repeat x-rays are in order. Occult fractures can occur in any of the carpal bones of the wrist, but the most common are the navicular (Figure 8-8), the pisiform or lunate, and the scaphoid. The usual history is a fall on the outstretched hand, complaints of tenderness, pain on motion, and swelling at the base of the thumb.

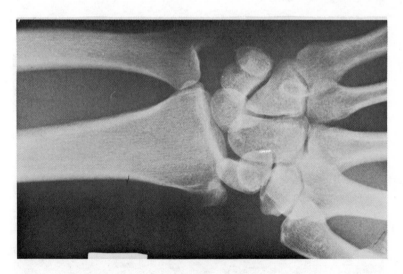

Figure 8-8 Delayed union of carpal navicular fracture.

Often, examination reveals minimal findings and there is usually no restriction of range of motion; x-rays are frequently negative. The injury is treated as a sprain and the wrist is immobilized. However, the patient does not improve, and pain persists at the base of the thumb. This patient should be x-rayed, as fracture lines may only become apparent after the passage of several days or longer. If a fracture is present, it is serious; such fractures heal only after immobilization for an extensive period of time, in some cases six to nine months. Immobilization is necessary in order to prevent a nonunion. If nonunion does occur, surgical correction is required to maintain the integrity of the wrist.

In the hand the carpal bone that is most frequently dislocated is the lunate (Figure 8-9). This also occurs on an outstretched hand in falling or stopping oneself, or even trying to catch a fast-moving object with an unprotected hand. It should be recognized early, and immobilized after reduction. If it is not recognized and the dislocation reduced, aseptic necrosis may occur necessitating surgical correction.

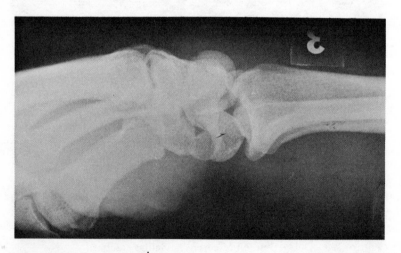

Figure 8-9 Posteroanterior view of wrist showing lunate dislocation and navicular fracture.

Both navicular and lunate injuries can produce prolonged disability. A carpal bone injury should always be suspected if an athlete does not respond to care and continues to have pain in the wrist or at the base of the thumb.

CONCLUSIONS

The arm plays a critical role in baseball and many other sports. The main sites of trauma are the shoulder girdle, elbow, wrist, and hand. The action of throwing is a very complex motion involving the entire body. Injuries are usually to soft tissues with bony and articular changes occurring later.

The musculotendinous structures are the main source of power in the throwing motion. Injuries occur to the shoulder by overstretching the muscle fibers or by violent muscular contraction. The nature of these injuries is modified by many things including: loose-tightness of the joints and musculature, the age of the athlete, the distance to be thrown, the presence of muscle weakness, fatigue, incoordination, and the amount of previous degenerative changes in the joint.

Accurate definition of the throwing motion allows coordination of the injury with its position in the phase of throwing as well as the anatomic location of the lesion on clinical examination. The most common throwing or circumduction injuries to the shoulder girdle were discussed because of the great importance of the throwing arm in sports.

Athletic lesions involving the elbow may be divided into two groups, the preadolescent and adolescent group and the adults. Injuries occur associated with various phases of pitching, throwing, racquet-hitting, etc. In the pitcher they result from stresses incurred primarily during the acceleration and follow-through phases.

Preseason conditioning should be a year-round program of stretching and conditioning to maintain flexibility and strength in the structures of the arm and entire body. Whether the athlete plays soccer, tennis, golf, basketball, or football, there are three basic components to preseason conditioning and injury prevention. First is maintenance of cardiovascular and pulmonary fitness. Second is a good flexibility and agility program. The third is a year-round weight-training program for strength, power, and speed.

It is extremely important for the physician to remember that the preadolescent and adolescent athletes are not miniature adults. They are not physically mature, and are not prepared to handle the demands, both physical and mental, that are commonplace for the adult involved in sports.

SUGGESTED READINGS

Adams, J.E. Bone injuries in very young athletes. *Clin Orthop.* 58:129–140, 1968.

Armstrong, J.R., and Tucker, W.E. (Eds.) *Injury in Sport: The Physiology, Prevention, and Treatment of Injuries Associated with Sport.* Springfield, Ill: Charles C Thomas, 1964, p. 153.

Brogdon, B.G., and Crow, N.E. Little Leaguer's elbow. *Am J Roentgenol.* 83:671–675, 1960.

Brown, R., Blazina, M.E., Kerlan, R.K., et al. Osteochondritis of the capitellum. *J Sports Med Phys Fitness.* 2:27–46, 1974.

Gugenheim, J.D., Jr., Stanley, R.F., Woods, G.W., et al. Little League survey: the Houston study. *Am J Sports Med.* 4:189–200, 1976.

Hale, C.J. Injuries among 711,810 Little League baseball players. *J Sports Med Phys Fitness.* 1:80–83, 1961.

Larson, R.L., Singer, K.M., Bergstom, R., et al. Little League survey: the Eugene study. *Am J Sports Med.* 4:201–209, 1976.

Lipscomb, A.B. Baseball pitching injuries in growing athletes. *J Sports Med Phys Fitness.* 3:25–34, 1975.

Middleman, I.C. Shoulder and elbow lesions of baseball players. *Am J Surg.* 102:627–632, 1961.

Smith, F.M. Medial epicondyle injuries. *JAMA.* 142:396–402, 1950.

Torg, J.S., Pollack, H., and Sweterlitsch, P. The effect of competitive pitching on the shoulders and elbows of preadolescent baseball players. *Pediatrics* 49:267–272, 1972.

Torg, J.S. Little League: "The theft of a carefree youth!" *Phys Sportsmed.* 1:72–78, 1973.

Tullos, H.S., and King, J.W. Lesions of the pitching arm in adolescents. *JAMA* 220:264–271, 1972.

9 The Prevention of Athletic Head and Spine Injuries

Robert C. Cantu, MD

The head and spine are unique in that their contents are incapable of regeneration. The brain and spinal cord cannot regrow lost cells, as can the other organs of the body, and thus injury to these structures takes on a singular importance. Many parts of the body are today capable of being replaced, either by artificial hardware or transplanted parts. The list is long, with virtually every major joint (ankle, knee, hip, elbow, shoulder) and most organs capable of replacement. The head and spine are not included because their contents cannot be transplanted. The most complex and vital area of the body, the central nervous system housed in the skull and spine, is capable of recovery from injury to cells, but once a cell or cells have died, no replacement is possible.

With these sobering facts in mind, Tables 9-1 and 9-2 list the most hazardous sports to the head and spine. In terms of injury prevention, perhaps one ought to start with considering avoiding these activities. Automobile racing is an example; one study showed 30% of new participants over a two-year period were either killed or so seriously injured they could not compete again.[1] Motor-(or as I prefer sui-)cycles, where 80% of the serious injuries befall those riding six months or less, are even more dangerous. In terms of the percentage of fatalities per participant, hang gliding ranks at the top. In this most dangerous of pursuits, the use of adequate helmets is not even uniformly seen.

Table 9-1
Sports of Maximal Risk to the Spine

Automobile racing
Diving
Football (only team sport)
Hang gliding
Motorcycle racing

Table 9-2
Sports with High Risk for Spine Injury

Gymnastics
Horseback riding
Mountain climbing
Parachuting
Ski jumping
Sky diving
Sky gliding
Snowmobiling
Trampolining

Football is the one team sport that makes it into the most hazardous head and spine injury group. This perhaps reflects more the severity of certain head and spine injuries, rather than the actual numbers. Although the data-gathering is far from precise, many large sports medicine services see more spine injuries from gymnastics than football.

In the last two decades, as football helmets were vastly improved and protective face masks added, the use of the head as a blocking and tackling weapon came into vogue. With professionals showing the way on television, our younger athletes followed, sometimes with catastrophic consequences. While the incidence of serious head injuries diminished with improved helmets, there was actually an increase in serious spine injuries (Tables 9-3 and 9-4) attributed to the use of spearing with the head.

Table 9-3
Cervical Spine Fracture-Dislocations 1971–1975

High school	182
College	64
Other	13
Total	259

Table 9-4
Permanent Quadriplegias 1971–1975

High school	77
College	18
Other	4
Total	99

Figures 9-1 and 9-2 illustrate the mechanism of spine injury with spearing. Note the gentle "S" shape curve of the neck in normal posture (Figure 9-1). Note how the spine becomes straight when the neck is flexed (Figure 9-2). With the vertebral bodies lined up straight, vertical impact forces are directly transmitted from one vertebra to the next, allowing for minimal dissipation of the impact forces to be absorbed by the muscles. If the impact force exceeds the strength of the bone, it compacts it at one or more levels causing a compression fracture. If the fractured vertebra malaligns and is driven back into the spinal cord, quadriplegia may result.

Tables 9-5, 9-6, and 9-7 show that it is when tackling with the head, especially in the open field where momentum is greatest, that most serious neck injuries occur.[2] The individual most susceptible is the small defensive back, often the fast but light safety, who attempts to bring down a larger, heavier back with a head tackle. Clearly, the high school athlete, where the degree of physical maturation and athletic ability has the greatest degree of variation, is at greatest risk.

Presently, catastrophic football head and neck injuries are at the lowest level in the last 18 years, approximately 0.5 per 100,000 athletes.[3] This represents an over 600% reduction from peak years in the later 1960s. It directly reflects the 1976 rule

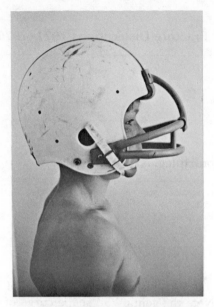

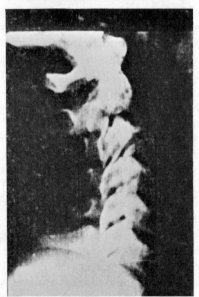

Figure 9-1 Normal "neutral" neck posture.

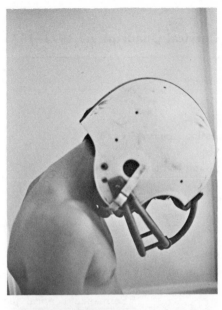

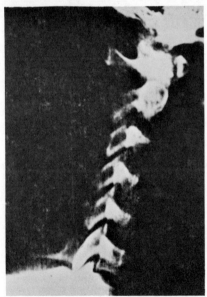

Figure 9-2 Flexed "spearing" neck posture.

Table 9-5
Permanent Cervical Quadriplegia 1971–1975

Mechanism of injury	No. of injuries
Hyperflexion	10
Hyperextension	3
Vertical compression (spearing)	52
Knee/thigh to head	15
Collision/pile/ground contact	11
Tackled	7
Machine-related	3
Face mask acting as lever	0

Table 9-6
Injuries by Position 1971–1975

	Permanent cervical quadriplegia (%)	
	High school	*College*
Defensive back	52	73
Linebacker	10	0
Specialty team	13	7
Offensive back	11	7
Defensive line	10	0
Offensive line	4	13

Table 9-7
Injury by Activity 1971–1975

	Permanent cervical quadriplegia (%)	
	High school	*College*
Tackling	72	78
Tackled	14	22
Blocking	6	0
Drill	3	0
Collision/pileup	3	0
Machine-related	2	0

change to prohibit butt blocking and face tackling, and also the football helmet standard established by the National Operating Committee on Standards for Athletic Equipment (NOCSAE). Improved conditioning programs, especially neck and back exercise programs, and improved supervision by team physicians and trainers, are other factors.

While football fatalities and catastrophic injuries will never be totally eliminated, their occurrence is now rare. Most entire football conferences go decades without such a problem, while yearly almost each participating school has one or more fatalities or catastrophic injuries attributed to a car or motorcycle accident. For the high school student, it is clearly more dangerous to drive a car or motorcycle than to play football.

The trend today is to treat and rehabilitate spinal injuries at regional centers. Many of these centers report diving accidents as the single most common cause of cervical spinal cord injury. In one ten-year period at Rancho Los Amigos Hospital, a regional spinal service for southwestern United States, over half of the 1600 patients admitted to the spinal-injury service with cervical cord impairment sustained the injury while diving.[4] Almost all of these injuries occurred not under conditions of competition or training, but during unsupervised recreation. The old adage, "look before you leap," could not be more pertinent as virtually all of these accidents involved diving into too-shallow water, and thus were preventable. Immaturity, impaired judgment, lack of education, training, and discipline are more important than the sport itself in these injuries.[5,6]

The following tips to avoid trouble in diving are derived from the Shields et al.[4]

1. Never dive into unfamiliar water.
2. Do not assume the water is deep enough. Even familiar lakes, rivers, and swimming holes change levels.
3. If you are present at a spinal cord injury, keep the victim's head and neck from bending and twisting.
4. Never dive near dredging or construction work. The water level may have dropped and dangerous objects may be just beneath the surface.

5. Do not drink before diving or swimming. Alcohol distorts judgment.
6. Water around a raft can be dangerous, especially if the water level is down. A slackened cable permits the raft to drift, putting the cable and anchor into the diving area.
7. Cloudy water can conceal hazardous objects. Check the bottom.

It was also of interest that during this same ten-year period the second most common cause of cervical cord injury was also a recreational water sport, surfing. Football ranked third, but was one-half that of surfing and less than one-fifth of those from diving. The message from the experience at Rancho Los Amigos is clear; 73% of cervical spinal cord injuries occurred in water-related sports, and almost all were preventable. Football cervical spinal cord injuries were less than one-fifth as common, but occurred even with the keenest of supervision.

The prevention of head injuries is essentially limited to using appropriate approved protective headgear such as the NOCSAE football helmet, then taking your chances. The brain cannot be preconditioned to accept trauma; in fact the opposite is true. If a young athlete has incurred more than one concussion in a given year, then contact sports should be avoided for the rest of that school year. This is even more cogently urged if a brain wave tracing (EEG) shows any abnormal slowing.

In contrast to the brain, the neck can be strengthened and in this manner injury risk lessened. Figures 9-3 and 9-4 depict two useful, safe exercises to strengthen neck muscles. They require no machines or fancy equipment, and when combined with appropriate warm-up and cool-off exercises, plus avoidance of the head as a battering ram, constitute the maximal active defense against serious cervical injury.

A few additional comments are appropriate regarding the prevention of neck injuries. Minor neurologic injuries can rapidly become major if neck injuries are not immediately detected. Such detection is not difficult in the conscious patient as he will describe neck pain and the neck muscles will go into spasm splinting a cervical fracture. This is not true for the unconscious

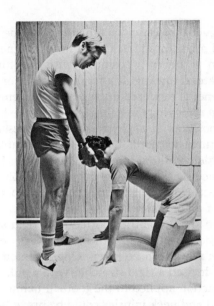

Figure 9-3   Neck flexion strengthening exercise.

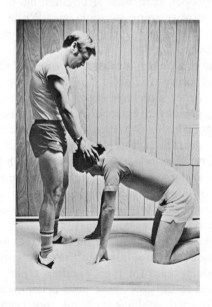

Figure 9-4   Neck extension strengthening exercise.

patient; thus every unconscious athlete should be handled as if he or she had a fractured neck. The head and neck should be maintained in a neutral position, with no forced flexion-extension or lateral turning. If a football player or other athlete wearing a helmet is rendered unconscious, extreme care should be exercised in removing the helmet, keeping the head and neck in a neutral position. If a physician is not present and if the athlete is breathing comfortably, it is often advisable to transport the injured athlete without removing the helmet. If breathing is labored, the face mask can be removed with bolt cutters, or in some cases a screwdriver, to gain access to the face and mouth for insertion of an oral airway.

The athlete should be transported on a rigid stretcher with the neck immobilized by a brace, sandbags, etc, until appropriate neck x-rays can be taken. One ingenious team physician has even devised a rigid stretcher with a pulley attachment for cervical traction applied to the football helmet.[6]

Many head and neck injuries could be prevented, or at least lessened, by proper care and strengthening of the cervical, thoracic, and lumbar spine musculature. While important for the head and neck, an appropriate exercise program is essential for the lower back.

At one time or another, almost everyone will experience low back pain.[7-10] A recent US Public Health Service report indicates that 70 million Americans have experienced at least one severe, incapacitating, prolonged episode of low back pain.[10] The National Center for Health Statistics states chronic and recurring back ailments form the largest single medical ailment.[10] Today, low back pain represents a major national health problem with over 15 billion dollars expended annually on the treatment and compensation of low back sufferers. In industry, compensation for low back problems represents a figure in excess of the cost of all other industrial injuries combined.[7]

Experience in sports medicine indicates that low back problems are a very common ailment in the athlete and nonathlete alike. The medical team for the Canadian athletes at the 1976 Olympic Games found low back pain a common problem in their highly trained athletes.[11] Many outstanding Olympic athletes tolerate low back pain as a constant recurring problem, and in some cases the disorder has progressed to the point of neurologic involvement with the athlete still competing.

What are the causes of low back pain? Why are young, vigorous, physically fit, elite male and female athletes suffering the same symptoms so prevalent in the unfit, sedentary middle-aged? The answers to these questions and the elimination of the problem require an understanding of the anatomy and pathology of low back pain.

ANATOMY OF THE LOW BACK

The lower back is composed of five mobile lumbar vertebrae with cartilaginous cushions (discs) between them, and the fused bones of the sacrum and coccyx, which form the back of the pelvis. There are also ligaments, thick dense tough strands of connective tissue, that attach one bone to another. These ligaments hold the foundation blocks of the low back, the vertebrae, sacrum, coccyx, and pelvis, together. All these ligaments have some elasticity and thus provide the back with mobility. The five major groups of ligaments of the low back and their mechanism of injury are listed.

Interspinal ligaments These ligaments extend from one spinous process to another and limit forward bending. They relax in extension and are torn or ruptured by extremes of forward bending (flexion).

Intertransverse ligaments These ligaments extend from one transverse process to another and limit sideward bending. They are torn or ruptured by extremes of sideward bending.

Ligamenta flava These form the roof of the spinal canal and bind rear segments of vertebrae. They are more elastic than other ligaments and are rarely torn.

Anterior and posterior longitudinal ligaments These run front (anterior) and back (posterior) along the longitudinal surface from one vertebra to another. They blend with and reinforce the annuli fibrosi. The anterior is much stronger than the posterior; the posterior disc ruptures more often than the anterior.

Annuli fibrosi disci intervertebralis These are the hard outer circumferential coverings of the nuclei pulposi or discs. The radial relationship of the fibers adds strength and has been copied by industry with the radial-ply tire. The annuli serve to restrict excessive motion between the vertebrae and to hold in place the nuclei pulposi (discs) with their resultant cushion effect.

The muscles of the back, abdomen, and hip are responsible for both support and movement of the back. There are four groups of muscles essential for support of the back that can play a major role in back pain. It is convenient to think of the low back as a pole held erect by four guy-wire muscle groups: the abdominal, the extensor, and the two sides.

Abdominal muscles These anterior guy wires are the rectus abdominus, internal oblique, external oblique, and transverse abdominus muscles. They extend from the rib cage to the sides and front of the pelvis where they attach by strong rough connective tissues called tendons. They support the abdominal cavity and control bending movements of the spine. When they are tensed, they relieve strain on the back. Investigators have demonstrated it is the strong abdominal muscles that allow one to lift weights that would otherwise crush the spine.

Extensor muscles These posterior guy wires consist of many layers, some spanning a single vertebra and others many, from the low back to the neck. Their tendons attach to the spine, pelvis, ribs, and head. These muscles are maximally used for pulling or pushing a heavy object. They are injured by posterior (arching) movements of the back.

Side muscles The two lateral guy wire groups control the sideward bending of the back by contraction of the quadratus lumborum and the psoas major. The psoas major is one of the body's largest muscles running from the side of the spine through the pelvis to attach to the anterior surface of the femur just below the hip joint.

These three groups of muscles, the abdominal, extensor, and two side muscles, constitute the four guy wires to support the back. However, the hips, by virtue of their relationship to the pelvis and thus the pelvis to the spine, can have a very significant effect on the back. Of the four hip muscle groups, the flexors (lift hips up), abductors (turn hips out), adductors (turn hips in), and extensors (lift hips back), the latter are the most massive and important to the back. The hip extensor muscles as a group control lumbar lordosis, a condition that when excessive is called "sway back" by the layperson and is a major cause of back pain. The hip extensors in combination with the hip flexors are essential in the maintenance of good posture.

Common Causes of Low Back Pain in the Athlete

Few athletic back injuries involve a ruptured disc or spine fracture. The definitive medical treatment of these disorders is beyond the scope of this book, but their early recognition and emergency care is vital and will be covered later.

Almost all athletic injuries to the low back involve either a contusion; a bruise from a direct blow; a sprain, a pulling with stretching and tearing of the muscles or their tendons; or a strain, tearing of a ligament. In general, a strain is most painful when the back is forced in the opposite direction, and a sprain produces pain when the affected muscle is contracted. From a practical standpoint due to the intricate relationships of the muscles, tendons, and ligaments of the back and the fact that most injuries involve two or all three entities, trying to separate them is academic.

The cause of most back strains and sprains in the athlete and nonathlete alike is weak muscles, especially the abdominal muscles and hip flexors, and tension or lack of flexibility, especially in the hamstring hip extensor muscles. But how could world-class athletes have weak muscles, you ask? Because during intensive training for the specific requirements of their sport, they neglect anatomic areas (the back-abdomen-hip) that do not seem to require development for success in their sport. At the 1976 Olympics, the Canadian medical team found the abdominal muscles underdeveloped in many world-class athletes.[11] Some of Canada's top athletes had trouble executing more than one or two bent-knee sit-ups. In general, athletes have strong extensor muscles (the back and hip), and the flexor muscles in one or both regions are frequently underdeveloped.

135

Mechanisms of Back Strain and Sprain

Most strains and sprains develop in one of two ways. The first is by a sudden, abrupt, violent extension contraction on an overloaded, unprepared, or underdeveloped spine, especially when there is some rotation in the attempted movement. This can result in stretching a few fibers, a complete tear, or an avulsion fracture of a spinous or transverse process.

The second mechanism involves a chronic strain, often with associated poor posture—excessive lumbar lordosis. Here there is a continuation of the underlying disease with recurring injury to the original and/or adjacent sites.

Through the repetition of training, many sports predispose to low back pain. Most sports involve either strong back extension movements, as opposed to strong flexion, or else external forces that produce extension. Track athletes run in forced extension. The discus thrower, shot putter, and weight lifter all propel heavy weights with the back extended. Gymnasts repeatedly dismount with a hyperextended low back as the feet hit the mat. So, too, the diver hits the water in extension with foot-entry dives.

EXAMINATION OF BACK INJURIES

Acute

For practical purposes, the back examination of an acutely injured athlete seen on the athletic field will be discussed separately from the ambulatory back-injured patient seen in the office or clinic. The essential medical equipment for this examination includes your hands, a pin, and a reflex hammer. Ice and/or ethylene chloride freezing spray, and a fracture board or rigid stretcher represent the primary "on the field" treatment aids.

When an athlete is stricken with a back injury during competition, whether it is after a tackle in football, a slide in baseball, a fall in basketball, or riding the pole vault pole back down to the ground as happened in one high school jumper who froze with the pole in his hands, the initial examination should

136

be on the spot. Although unstable fractures and fracture-dislocations with and without neurologic involvement are uncommon in the low back, a careful examination to eliminate their presence is essential as suspicion alone dictates great care in transport. When one arrives at the side of the conscious injured athlete, the first question asked is where does it hurt. For the back-injured athlete, even before examining his back, the next question is whether any loss of feeling or numbness or weakness is appreciated in the lower extremities. The spinal cord ends at the lower border of the first lumbar vertebra in most adults. Injury to the spinal cord usually implies a fracture-dislocation or dislocation of the vertebra at the instant of impact with spontaneous relocation. Both should be considered unstable and the athlete transported off the field and to a hospital on a fracture board.

Injury to the spinal cord may produce either complete or incomplete loss of function of the nervous system below the level of the lesion. In a complete lesion, sensation, motor power, and reflexes in the legs are lost as well as bowel and bladder control. In an incomplete lesion, varying degrees of these functions are retained. The seriousness of either a complete or incomplete lesion of the spinal cord renders essential a neurologic evaluation of sensation, movement, and knee and ankle reflexes as soon as the patient is seen. If any neurologic deficit is recorded, then the patient must be transported from the field on a fracture board.

Fortunately, few back injuries have neurologic impairment. Having determined there is none, now the back muscles themselves should be examined. Palpation of the back should start in the midline with a thumb pressing over each spinous process. Exquisite pain over one spinous process suggests a possible fracture or tear of the interspinal ligaments. Such a fracture rarely has associated vertebral instability. Pain described as deep in the back with localized tenderness either over one or in between two spinous processes raises suspicion for a compression fracture of a vertebra. Most compression fractures involve either the 11th or 12th dorsal vertebra or one of the first two lumbar vertebrae. The young pole vaulter mentioned above who did not let go of his pole and rode it back down incurred a fracture-dislocation of the first and second lumbar vertebrae. While most compression fractures, like spinous or transverse process fractures, are stable, if suspected due to focal midline tenderness on palpation, it is wisest to transport the injured athlete on a fracture board until such time as x-rays clearly establish the fracture is stable. The definitive treatment of these fractures and their complications, from paralytic ileus, to neurologic deficit, to decubitus ulcers is beyond the intent of this chapter.

Now having eliminated the most worrisome back injuries as will usually be the case, continue to palpate the back paraspinal muscles; also continue around the abdominal wall being certain to include the side flexor and rotator muscles. Areas of focal tenderness may be found that indicate local spasm. If a large swelling is present, this usually represents a contusion with hemorrhage into the muscle. A slight swelling could indicate contusion, strain, sprain, or any combination thereof. The immediate treatment is application of cold to the trigger point, either by an ice pack or freezing spray. Later treatment will involve heat, rest, and analgesic and antiinflammatory medication. In virtually all of these injuries, the athlete can safely walk from the field under his own power.

Nonacute

A small percentage of athletes with low back problems will not only have low back pain, but also pain that radiates from the back into the buttock and/or down one or both legs. Coughing, sneezing, straining to pass urine or at bowel movements usually makes the leg pain worse. Numbness may also be felt, usually in the foot either over the medial half or along the lateral side. This pattern of pain is called sciatica and suggests that a ruptured disc is pressing on a nerve root. Discs are the fibrocartilaginous cushions between the vertebrae. As the body ages the discs lose fluid content, becoming slightly narrower, causing a slight shrinkage in height. The outer more fibrous capsule of the disc, called the annulus fibrosus, may also tear, allowing the disc to rupture posteriorly out of the disc space and compress the nerve root as it exits from the spine. Most simple ruptures can be treated successfully with a period of bedrest, muscle relaxants, antiinflammatory medicines, analgesics, and later, exercises. A minor percentage with neurologic deficit, ie, a reflex absence at knee or ankle, weakness of ankle or great toe extension, or persistent pain and numbness, will require surgical excision of the ruptured disc. With careful selection, the success of such surgery should exceed 90%. Following surgery, the athlete should adhere to the exercises and advice given in this chapter and should be able to resume competition.

A third group of athletes with low back problems suffer from mechanical misalignment of the vertebrae—spondylolisthesis. This diagnosis is established by x-ray of the back. If there is instability documented by further misalignment as the back is placed through flexion and extension maneuvers, then a surgical procedure of lumbar fusion may be indicated.[12,13] An abnormal lateral curvature of the spine (scoliosis) is yet another cause of low back pain. If severe in children, this may require surgical correction that is a very extensive and time-consuming procedure. Severe scoliosis renders athletic excellence very remote. The mild form seen in some athletes can be pain-free if the exercises and hints in this chapter are followed. Only a physician and especially an orthopedist or neurosurgeon is properly qualified to evaluate and treat the athlete's low back problem. Thus, the exercises and advice in this chapter are primarily directed at the athlete with low back pain but without neurologic deficit, or who has already had concern for a ruptured disc or spinal instability eliminated by appropriate medical consultation.

The vast majority of athletes with low back pain will have no neurologic symptoms, deficits, or spinal instability. Palpation, as with the acute injury of the paraspinal, side flexor and rotator, and abdominal muscles, usually reveals segmental spasm, tenderness, or an area of point tenderness.

Athletes are usually thin, quite physically fit, but have an accentuated lumbar lordosis when walking. The posterior erector spinal muscles are strong, but the abdominal (flexor) muscles, although flat, in comparison are quite weak. A good test of abdominal muscle strength is a slow bent-knee sit-up. An athlete should be able to do 20 or more, but some Olympic-class athletes with back problems have trouble doing one.[11] The back extensor muscles are tested with the athlete on his abdomen with a pillow under the hips as a cushion. To test the upper back, with the hands behind the head, raise elbows, chin, and trunk off the floor as long as possible (Figure 9-5). Low back strength is tested by keeping the head down with hands behind while both legs held together with knees straight are raised off the floor (Figure 9-6). In both exercises, 20 seconds indicates strong muscles and under 10 weak.

Frequently, back rotation is weak. When the overdeveloped extensors are tight, both flexion and rotation are compromised. In some athletes, the hip flexor and hamstring muscles will be tight. In such cases, one cannot touch the floor with fingertips with the knees straight (Figure 9-7). Ideally, the hamstring muscles should be at least 60% to 80% as strong as the quadriceps; the closer to 80% the fewer back problems encountered. To test the strength of the hip flexor muscles, have the athlete lie on his back, legs extended, hands clasped behind the head. With legs touching, have him left his feet about 10 inches off the floor and hold this position for as long as possible. Over 20 seconds indicates strong muscles, under 10 quite weak hip flexor muscles (Figure 9-8).

TREATMENT

The successful treatment of low back pain in athletes involves a three-step program. First is the relief of pain and spasm; second, the adoption of an appropriate exercise program that includes both stretching and strengthening exercises; third, an educational program that takes into consideration one's training program and is tailored to preventing future injuries.

Relief of Pain and Spasm

Ice, analgesics, muscle relaxants, antiinflammatory agents, and rest are used in the acute stages while heat, muscle stimulation, and/or ultrasound, physical therapy, and the same pharmacologic agents are used 12 or more hours after injury. Ultrasound and gentle muscle stimulation seem to more rapidly dissipate

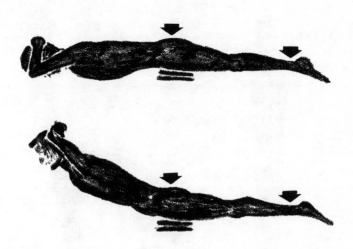

Figure 9-5 Test for upper back strength.

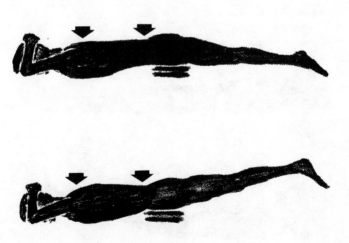

Figure 9-6 Test for lower back strength.

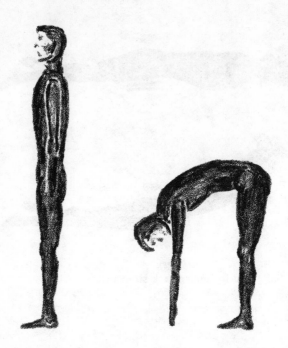

Figure 9-7 Test for tight hip flexor and hamstring muscles.

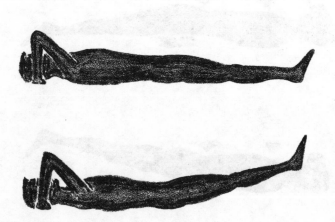

Figure 9-8 Test for hip flexor strength.

muscle spasm, point tenderness, and general soreness. This is probably due to enhanced muscle circulation and exchange at the cellular level of prescribed pharmacologic agents plus elimination of toxic cellular products.[14] Actually, while modes of pain relief exist, no one treatment has been clearly demonstrated to accelerate actual tissue healing.

Stretching and Strengthening Exercises

Medications, manipulations, massage, ultrasound, and hot and cold applications do not strengthen a weakened or compromised part of the body. Low back pain is usually due to muscles that are weak, tense, fatigued, or all three. Once the healing process has occurred, it is essential to embark on an exercise program to rebuild the back and abdominal musculature.

Before the strengthening exercises are commenced, it is important first to have executed specific stretching exercises for the lumbar extensor and pelvic rotator, hip flexor, and hamstring and hip extensor muscles.

Stretching   Athletes can stretch their lower back muscles by lying on a mat and bringing the feet up over the face to touch extended toes beyond the head (Figure 9-9). It is important that these movements are executed fluidly with no sudden jerking. A good exercise to stretch the hip flexor muscles is shown in Figure 9-10. The athlete lies on his back, knees bent, feet under the buttocks. Then the arms reach as far toward the knees as possible as the back arches and the hips are thus maximally extended. The straight leg raise (Figure 9-11) and standing with one leg on waist-high table, nose-toe touch (Figure 9-12) are good flexibility exercises for the hamstrings; while the single knee raise and double knee hug (Figures 9-13 and 9-14) stretch the hamstrings, low back, and hip extensors. The athlete must work daily on flexibility exercises to maintain a good range of motion. They should become a routine part of his daily warm-up and cool-off exercises.

Strengthening   Exercises that strengthen the low back and abdominal muscles include some of the same exercises that stretch the hamstring and hip flexor muscles. Ten such exercises will now be presented. The exercises should be carried out on a hard, flat surface with adequate padding. A tumbling mat is ideal, but a thick rug with underpadding may suffice. For those exercises done supine, most find a small pillow placed under the neck will provide more comfort. One should wear loose, unrestrictive clothing. As mentioned previously, the exercises must always be initiated slowly to allow muscles to loosen up gradually. At no time employ jerking or snapping movements. Most find relaxing before exercising beneficial, and that heat treatment to the low back aids in loosening tight muscles. Slight

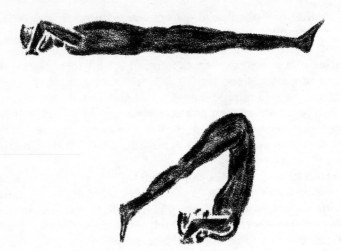

Figure 9-9 Exercise to stretch lower back muscles.

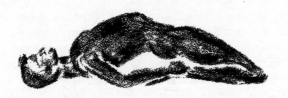

Figure 9-10 Exercise to stretch hip flexor muscles.

144

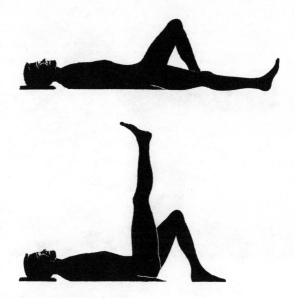

Figure 9-11 Straight leg raise.

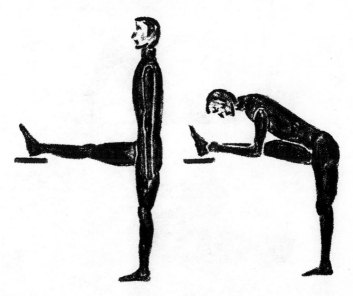

Figure 9-12 Exercise to stretch hamstring muscles.

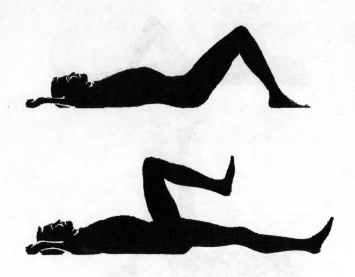

Figure 9-13 Single knee raise.

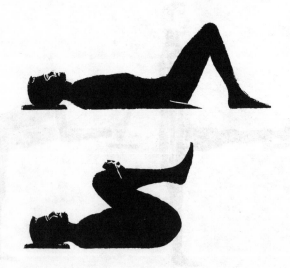

Figure 9-14 Double knee hug.

discomfort may occur as the exercises are performed, but if frank pain is experienced, the exercise period should be terminated. The exercises should be done daily, ideally twice a day in the beginning. Each athlete should progress at his own pace. Initially, five repetitions usually will suffice; then one can add a repetition or two daily to each exercise that can be accomplished with relative ease. If one or more of the exercises results in appreciable discomfort, then it should be abandoned while the remainder are continued. Only resume an exercise when it can be done without discomfort.

1. The back flattener (Figure 9-15) is to strengthen gluteal (buttock) and abdominal muscles and flatten the low back in lumbar lordosis. Lie on back on padded floor with knees well bent. Relax with arms above head. A small pillow may be placed under head if desired. Squeeze buttocks together as if trying to hold a piece of paper between them. At the same time, suck in and tighten the muscles of the abdomen. The back should flatten against the floor. This is the flat back position. Hold this position for a count of ten (10 seconds), relax and repeat the exercise three times in the beginning. Gradually attempt to increase to 20 repetitions.

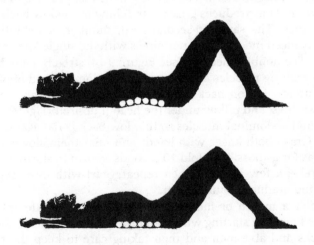

Figure 9-15 Back flattener.

After the basic exercise has been done for a week or more, additional flattening can be achieved by doing the exercise with the buttocks slightly raised (1 to 2 inches) off the floor at the time the buttocks are squeezed and abdomen tensed. Hold for the count of ten, relax, and repeat.

After several weeks of the basic exercise, gradually do the exercise with the knees less and less bent, until the exercise is executed with legs straight. The buttock raise need not be combined with this modification.

2. The single knee raise (see Figure 9-13) stretches low back, hip flexor, and hamstring (posterior thigh) muscles. Lie on back on a padded floor with arms above head and knees bent. Tighten buttocks and abdominal muscles as in exercise No. 1. Then raise one knee over chest toward chin as far as possible, hold for 10 seconds, return to starting position, and relax a few seconds before repeating with the opposite leg. Start with three repetitions of each knee, gradually advancing to ten.

3. The single knee hug (Figure 9-16) has the same purpose and is essentially the same exercise as the single knee raise, except the hands are not placed above the head, but rather are placed around the knee to be raised. The arms are used to pull (raise) the knee higher over the chest than was possible in exercise No. 2. This produces greater stretching of the low back and hamstrings. The same 10-second hold, number of repetitions, and advanced modification pertain as with the single knee raise.

4. The double knee hug (see Figure 9-14) stretches low back and hamstring muscles and strengthens abdominal and hip flexing muscles. Lie on back on a covered floor with knees bent, arms at sides, and pillow under the head if desired. Tighten buttocks and abdominal muscles so that low back is flat against the floor. Grasp both knees with hands and raise them slowly over chest as far as possible. Hold 10 seconds, return to starting position, relax a few seconds, then repeat. Start with three repetitions and gradually build to ten.

After a month or more of the basic exercise, attempt the double knee hug starting with both legs extended straight. Tense buttocks and abdomen and then taking care to keep the back flat, bend both knees, grasp knees with hands and raise over chest, hold 10 seconds and return to starting position to relax

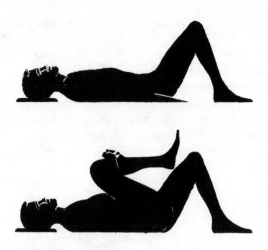

Figure 9-16 Single knee hug.

before repeating. The low back tends to arch when lifting and lowering the knee. If this cannot be done with the back against the floor, the athlete is not ready for this modification and should resume the basic knees-bent position. This extended-leg starting position strengthens both the hip flexing and abdominal muscles.

5. The single leg raise (see Figure 9-11) also stretches low back and hamstring muscles, and strengthens abdominal and hip-flexing muscles. Lie on back on a covered floor with one knee bent and one leg straight, arms at sides and a pillow under the head if desired. Tighten buttocks and abdominal muscles, then slowly raise the straight leg, keeping it straight and the back flat. Raise the leg as far as comfortably possible, then slowly lower the leg to the floor, keeping it straight and the back flat. Relax a few seconds and then repeat with the other leg. Start with three repetitions of each leg and gradually increase to ten.

After a month or more, attempt the single leg raise starting with both legs extended straight. Tense buttocks and low back and with back flat and legs out straight, raise one leg up as far as possible. As the leg is raised, back may not remain flat. Check this by using hand to see if back lifts from the floor when the leg is lifted and lowered. If it does, resume the basic exercise with one knee bent.

6. The partial sit-up (Figure 9-17) strengthens low back and abdominal muscles. Lie on back on a covered floor with knees well bent. Squeeze buttocks and tighten abdominal muscles; with low back on the floor, slowly raise head, neck, and lastly shoulders while extending arms to knees. Keep low back flat on the floor. Hold this position 10 seconds, return to starting position, rest a few seconds, and repeat. Start with three repetitions and progress to at least ten.

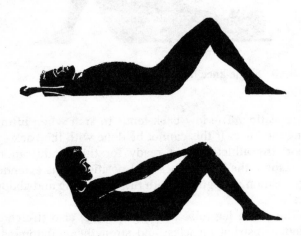

Figure 9-17 Partial sit-up.

After having progressed to ten repetitions, begin to progressively lift head and shoulders farther from the floor. The back will now lift off the floor. Keep knees bent. In the beginning, it may help to place feet under a heavy chair or some other restraint. Once abdominal muscles are strong enough, this should not be necessary and not done as this action actually allows the legs to help the abdomen in raising the body. The motion should be a gentle, smooth curling and uncurling. Never jerk to achieve greater height or an additional repetition and never strain or exert beyond reasonable comfort. Again, start with three repetitions and progress to at least ten.

7. Advanced sit-up (Figure 9-18) is used to maximally strengthen low back and abdominal muscles. Lie on back on a covered floor with knees well bent. Squeeze buttocks and tighten abdominal muscles. Start with arms folded over waist and lift head, shoulders, and back smoothly up to the position where arms are touching knees. Hold 10 seconds, return to the starting position, relax a few seconds and then repeat. Again, start with three repetitions and progress to at least ten.

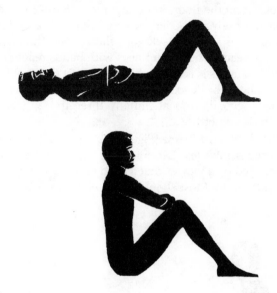

Figure 9-18 Advanced sit-up.

Progress gradually until ten of the basic advanced sit-ups can be easily and comfortably executed. Then try folding the arms in front of face instead of waist. Curl up to knees, hold 10 seconds, then return to the starting position, relax a few seconds and repeat. Start with three regpetitions. When this modified version can be accomplished ten times, a sit-up with hands clasped behind the head can be attempted. When this version can also be done ten times, attempt the most maximal version of a sit-up. This involves lying on the back on a padded inclined surface (ie, a tilt board with the foot end elevated). Knees should be bent as always, then with hands clasped behind neck, slowly and carefully execute the sit-up, hold 10 seconds, slowly uncurl to the starting position, relax, and repeat. This last version is clearly optional. The more inclined the board, the greater strength and effort will be required of your back and abdomen to accomplish the sit-up.

8. The sitting bend (Figure 9-19) strengthens the low back while stretching low back and hamstring muscles. Sit on a hard chair, feet flat on the floor, knees not more than 12 inches apart, arms folded loosely in the lap. Squeeze buttocks and tighten abdominal muscles so that back goes flat against the chair. Bend over, letting head go between knees with hands reaching for the floor. Bend as far as is comfortable, hold for a count of five, then slowly pull body back to the flat back sitting starting position. Relax a few seconds, repeat initially three times, gradually increasing to ten repetitions.

9. The deep knee bend (Figure 9-20) strengthens hamstring and quadriceps muscles. Do not begin this exercise until it has been confirmed by a viewer that a good back flattener (No. 1) has been accomplished. Most should not attempt this exercise until a

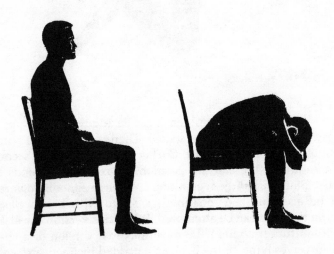

Figure 9-19 Sitting bend.

month into the exercise program. Discontinue this exercise if there is considerable lasting discomfort in your knees or hips.

Stand behind a sofa, desk, heavy chair, or similar structure holding onto it for balance. Squeeze and tighten buttocks and abdomen. Slowly bend knees and with a flat back, squat down as far as is reasonably comfortable, stop, stand up using only legs, and not arms. Relax for a second or two and repeat initially three times and gradually build up to ten repetitions.

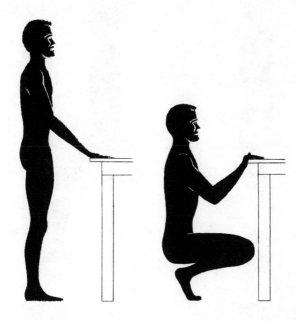

Figure 9-20   Deep knee bend.

10. Posture check (Figure 9-21) helps correct standing and walking. It also determines if the exercise program is accomplishing its goals.

Stand with back to the wall, pressing heels, buttocks, shoulders, and head against the wall. There should be no space between low back and the wall; if there is, the back is too arched and not flat. Move feet forward, bending knees so back slides a few inches down the wall. Now again, squeeze buttocks and tighten abdominal muscles, flattening lower back against the wall. While holding this position, walk feet back so as to slide up the wall. Standing straight, walk away from the wall and around the room. Return to the wall and back up to it to be certain that the proper posture was kept.

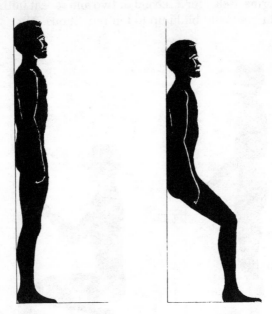

Figure 9-21 Posture check.

Educational Program

The final link in the low back pain elimination triangle involves educating the athlete how to avoid back problems, both in training and daily life. As previously mentioned, good posture is achieved by rotating the top of the pelvis backward, which flattens the curve in the low back. Common everyday tips to avoid the occurrence of low back pain include the following.

Standing and walking   Stand with lower back erect and as flat as possible. By squeezing buttocks and sucking in and tensing abdomen, the lower back is straightened. Walk, stand, and sit as tall as possible.

Bend knees when leaning, as when over a wash basin. Avoid leaning whenever possible and squat with a straight lower back.

Avoid high heeled shoes. They shorten Achilles tendons and increase lordosis.

Avoid standing for long periods of time, but if it is necessary, alternate leaning on the left foot and right foot, and if possible use the bent knee position as on a stool. This flattens the lower back.

When standing, do not lean back and support body with hands. Keep hands in front of body and lean forward slightly.

When turning to walk from a standing position, move feet first and then the body.

Open doors wide enough to walk through comfortably.

Carefully judge the height of curbs before stepping up or down.

Sitting Sit so that lower back is flat or slightly rounded outward, never with a forward curve.

Sit so that knees are higher than hips; this may require a small footstool for a short person in a high chair.

Hard seat backs that begin contact with back 4 to 6 inches above the seat and provide a flat support throughout the entire lumbar area are preferable.

Do not sit in a soft or overstuffed chair or sofa.

Avoid sitting in swivel chairs or chairs on rollers.

Do not sit with legs out straight on an ottoman or footstool.

Never sit in the same position for prolonged periods, get up and move around.

Driving Push front seat forward so that knees will be higher than hips and the pedals are easily reached without stretching.

Sit back with back flat, do not lean forward, sit tall.

Add a flat back rest if car seat is soft or if travelling a long distance.

If on a long trip, stop every 30 to 60 minutes, get out of car and walk about, tensing buttocks and abdomen to flatten the back for several minutes.

Always fasten seatbelt and shoulder harness.

Be sure car seat has a properly adjusted headrest.

Bedrest   Sleep or rest only on a flat firm mattress. If one is not available, place a bedboard of no less than three-quarter inch plywood under the mattress. A board of less thickness will sag, preventing proper spine alignment.

When sleeping, the preferred position is on the side, both arms in front, and knees slightly drawn up toward chin.

Do not sleep on stomach.

When lying on back, place a pillow under knees, as raising the legs flattens the lumbar curve.

When lying in bed, do not extend arms above head, relax them at sides.

If the doctor prescribes absolute bedrest, stay in bed. Raising body or twisting and turning can strain the back.

Sleep alone or in an oversized bed.

When getting out of bed, turn over on side, draw up knees, then swing legs over the side of the bed.

Lifting   When lifting, let the legs do the work, using the large muscles of the thighs instead of the small muscles of the back.

Do not twist the body, face the object.

Never lift with legs straight.

Do not lift heavy objects from car trunks.

Do not lift from a bending-forward position.

Do not reach over furniture to open and close windows.

Tuck in the buttocks and pull in the abdomen when lifting.

Only lift holding the object close to body.

Lift a heavy load no higher than the waist, and a light load no higher than the shoulders, as greater height increases lumbar lordosis.

To turn while lifting, pivot feet turning the whole body at one time.

In training, to minimize back injuries, the athlete should always warm up slowly and cool down after the main workout. Both the warm-up and cool-off periods should include back-stretching exercises. Calisthenics that involve hyperextension of the back such as back bends, straight leg sit-ups, or straight leg raises should be avoided when possible.

By faithfully carrying out a daily program of back exercise, the athlete can pursue a variety of potentially hazardous sports with minimal risk of back injury.

SPORTS MOST HAZARDOUS TO THE BACK

As discussed previously, most back injuries are sustained by acute hyperextension of the back. Football is felt by some to be legalized assault, often between physical unequals. It is one of the most hazardous sports to the body, and to the back in particular. This is especially true for the interior linemen (defensive ends, guards, tackles, and centers). A report from a major university with a recent number-one national ranking cited the fact that during one year, 50% of interior linemen sought medical attention for low back pain.[15] This report postulated biochemics of the back injury. As the lineman drives forward attempting to push the opponent backward, the lumbar spine is extended and this converts more of the force to a shearing force that can lead to pars interarticularis injury. It concluded that the high incidence of spondylolysis and spondylolisthesis seen in interior linemen is the result of repeated forces being transmitted to the pars interarticularis while players are in the lumbar-extended posture.

Weightlifting is another high-risk back-injury sport. This is especially true for the overhead military press, and the clean and jerk. Severe lordotic postures are also assumed when spiking a volleyball, hitting a twist serve or deep overhead stroke in tennis, putting the shot, throwing the discus or hammer, or even stretching for the tape in track. Extreme backward arching movements are required by the gymnast (especially in dismounts), diver, trampolinist, and squash, soccer, handball, and racquetball enthusiast. Also, sledding, downhill skiing, and snow and water ski jumping can result in excessive stresses to the low back. Both the hang glider and pole vaulter occasionally have precipitous descents in awkward postures that can result in back strain or even compression fractures.

Sports that are less likely to result in back injury include baseball, basketball, bowling, golf, figure skating, softball, ping-pong, water skiing, canoeing, rowing, fencing, cross-country skiing, badminton, and archery. Sports least likely to result in back injury include bicycling, hiking, swimming, fishing, curling, darts, skin diving, boccie, billiards, pool, and sailing.

As emphatically repeated throughout this chapter, the athlete can best prevent head and spine injuries by using approved headgear, appropriate techniques, and the daily execution of appropriate muscle stretching and strengthening exercises. For any sport, the athlete should always warm up slowly and include stretching exercises. In some sports, the most hazardous maneuvers can be modified. The serve, for example, and the overhead are the two tennis strokes most strenuous to the back. By tossing a serve slightly forward, less back extension is required and, thus, less back strain. For those who play a serve and volley game, it will also aid in gaining forward momentum toward the net. So, too, when hitting the overhead, go up to the ball hitting it slightly in front of the body. When trying for a low ball, whether tennis, handball, volleyball, softball, baseball, etc, whenever possible bend the knees rather than the back. Most gymnastic sports, including diving, stress good posture. The athlete at all times should sit and stand as tall as possible. The runner, equestrian, diver, and gymnast should keep the low back flat by tensing the buttocks and abdominal muscles whenever possible.

Thus, intelligently pursued and with adequate protection and preparation, the athlete can play a variety of potentially hazardous sports with little risk of injury. There is no substitution for the faithful daily execution of an appropriate exercise program, and the head must never be employed as a battering ram. The ultimate responsibility for avoiding head and spine injuries lies with the athlete himself or herself and the coaches and trainers who advise them.

REFERENCES

1. Bodnar, L.M. Sports medicine with reference to back and neck injuries. *Curr Pract Orthop Surg.* 7:116–153, 1977.

2. Torg, J.S., Quedenfeld, T.C., Burstein, A., et al. National football head and neck injury registry: report on cervical quadriplegia. *Am J Sports Med.* 7:127–132, 1979.

3. Mueller, F.O., and Blyth, C.S. Catastrophic head and neck injuries. *Phys Sportsmed.* 7:71–74, 1979.

4. Shields, C.L., Jr, Fox, J.M., and Stauffer, E.S. Cervical cord injuries in sports. *Phys Sportsmed.* 6:71–76, 1978.

5. Hubbard, D.D. Injuries to the spine in children and adolescents. *Clin Orthop.* 100:56–65, 1974.

6. Keweramini, L.S., and Taylor, R.G. Injuries to the cervical spine from diving accidents. *J Trauma.* 15:130–142, 1975.

7. Friedmann, L.W., and Galton, L. *Freedom from Backaches.* New York: Pocket Books, 1973.

8. Jones, L. *The Postural Complex.* Springfield, Ill: Charles C Thomas, 1955.

9. Kraus, H. *Backache Stress and Tension.* New York: Simon and Schuster, 1965.

10. Root, L., and Kiernan, T. *Oh, My Aching Back.* New York: New American Library, 1975.

11. Smith, C.F. Physical management of muscular low back pain in the athlete. *Can Med Assoc J.* 177:632–635, 1977.

12. Wiltse, L.L. Etiology of spondylolisthesis. *Clin Orthop.* 10:48–60, 1957.

13. Wiltse, L.L. Spondylolisthesis: classification and etiology. In *American Academy of Orthopedic Surgeons Symposium on the Spine.* St Louis: C.V. Mosby, 1969.

14. Harris, W.D. Low back pain in sports medicine. *J Arkansas Med Soc.* 74:377–379, 1978.

15. Ferguson, R.J. Low back pain in college football linemen. *J Sports Med Phys Fitness.* 2:63–80, 1974.

10 Panel Discussion

Robert C. Cantu, MD

Question: Can the athlete convert fast-twitch to slow-twitch fibers?

Dr Arnot: Yes, you can change the ability of fast-twitch fibers to do endurance work and endurance fibers to do sprint work, but you cannot change the actual proportions. The area that they occupy can be increased, however. By making fast-twitch fibers bigger and bigger they might occupy 90% of your muscle volume, even though only 60% of the fibers are of that type.

Q: Is it feasible to prescribe 65% to 85% of maximum predicted heart rate working with individuals 30 to 60 years old?

Dr Childs: Yes, depending on the age of the person. I advise people in general to get into the age-adjusted 75% to 80% area as routine performance. How fast they get into this depends on the condition they are in in the first place and how hard they push themselves. Depending on age and all other risk factors we have talked about, one adjusts this pace and is sensible about it. I have had no problems with that whatsoever. I think it is just a matter of safe, steady, careful progress.

Q: Can too much vitamin C be toxic?

Dr Cantu: Yes, there are toxic levels, approximately 4 to 5 gm or more per day. Most of us in the drugstore will see the supplement tablet being 250 mg; the highest I have seen is 500 mg. Thus we are talking in terms of taking 8 to 10 or more of those huge capsules per day. The toxic effects are primarily on the kidney, with stones being the major complication. It is a tremendously excessive amount.

Q: Do we abuse the body's musculoskeletal system by running?

Dr. Cantu: Excluding our brain, the only way we can retard the normal degenerative process of our ligaments, tendons, muscles, and bones is to stress them. I am not talking about super maximal amounts; I am not talking about pushing oneself beyond what is reasonable. The evidence is clear that the way you retard degenerative conditions of those tissues is to use them. Consequently, while jogging is an excellent manner of obtaining cardiopulmonary fitness and lower extremity fitness, total fitness will require additional exercise for your upper body: calesthenics, repetitive use of light weights, etc. Running and jogging alone will not make the whole body totally fit.

Q: Why are ECG stress tests not giving the accurate results originally predicted?

Dr Childs: In most situations they are. However, we now realize that false-positives and -negatives are seen. What are we doing when we give a person an ECG stress test? We put a person either on a bicycle or treadmill and exercise him at steadily accelerating work levels achieving progressively increasing heart rates while monitoring with a continuous ECG to establish signs or changes that are held to indicate coronary artery disease. In some studies the incidence of false-positives was discouragingly high. For the person who is trying to introduce the general population to an aerobic exercise program this presents a real dilemma. What is the best thing to do? I asked this very question myself of Dr Ellestad at a recent conference; what I asked him specifically was, given a person on whom you have done a careful history and physical exam, there are no symptoms, the family history is good, there is no hyperlipidemia—in other words, you do not see significant risk factors—is a stress test necessary? His answer was no. During the course of an exercise program a person should know what to look for in terms of symptoms, chest pain, palpitations, etc that should encourage him to call the doctor and have a stress ECG. As a blanket rule I must say, especially for most women before the menopause where the incidence of coronary artery disease is very low, a stress ECG is not necessary.

Q: When you exercise near busy roadways does the polluted air increase pulmonary disease and are the pollutants readily extracted?

Dr Arnot: I would like to specifically comment on carbon monoxide. A very small percentage of carbon monoxide in the air will affect athletic performance. It is at the level of 10% of carbon monoxide in our blood by volume that we start to get symptoms, lethargy and headache especially. At high exercise rates there is a tremendous amount of air moving through the lung and tissue metabolic demands are high; thus a very small amount of carbon monoxide will result in decreased physical performance. It turns out that as low as 5 to 10 parts per million will give an individual symptoms of carbon monoxide poisoning when they are at a very severe exercise level. So, the answer to this question is yes; if you are on an open roadway you will be extracting a fair amount of carbon monoxide and may actually find a deterioration in performance. Dr George Sheehan, who does quite a bit of writing about running, recommends if you are racing stay in the outside lane, if you pass any trucks stay well back of any that has any big exhaust and if you have a chance, pass.

Q: Please comment on the use of diet pills.

Dr Childs: There is really not much one can say favorably as I look at it. The reason should be clear from what I had to say earlier. I really feel very strongly that the emphasis should not be just on losing weight but rather body fat. As far as the diet pills go, diethylpropion (Tenuate) is one of a small number of pills that is responsibly used in some carefully selected cases to-day. There are all kinds of other things that are used for pills today, from the harmless but relatively ineffective cellulose compounds to the other extremes of amphetamines, thyroid hormone, and diuretics. These compounds are being used to achieve a quick result but can have long-term deleterious effects on the person using them. I would say there is a place for a few so-called diet pills under certain, carefully controlled circumstances, but there is no place for most.

Q: Is there a safe, quick way for a 17-year-old wrestler to lose 13 to 15 lb?

Dr Cantu: No! And, what is more, hopefully there is going to be strict enforcement of what has previously been very common practice in wrestlers, of high school, collegiate, and even Olympic caliber. That is, actually wrestling matches at a weight many pounds in excess of what they weigh in at. As if they got into a pressure cooker and sweated off 15 lb to take their 200 lb down to 180 lb to get into a different weight classification. No, there is no quick, safe way to lose 13 to 15 lb. You have to lose water to do that and with that electrolytes are lost and that is not safe and very much to be discouraged.

Q: My wife supports my running but is not interested in running herself. Her position is that she does not need exercise, that she gets enough just walking through the school during the day—is she correct in her assessment?

Dr Childs: I think you already know the answer to that in terms of what we have discussed. We are advocating aerobic exercise training, nonintermittent exercise at levels that increase the heart rate 60% to 80% of maximum. I must say, husbands and wives are almost universally unsuccessful in convincing each other that this is the way to go. I usually will ask husbands and wives, if they are going to do the same exercise form together, not to insist on doing it neck and neck because of the inevitable differences in performance and bad vibes that arise. I would say the thing that often is successful in getting one's spouse to get going where you already are, is not the, "gee, you ought to do this" which gets interpreted as "I'm bad because I don't," but the "gee, I love you, I'm fond of you, I would love to see you in great shape so that you can stick around and be in the family for more years. Also so that we and the kids can have more fun together, and remember that time that everybody pooped out on Mt Monadnock." In other words, if it is put in terms of one's own wishes and hopes in a positive sense it will often get better results. Otherwise, unfortunately it does often get misinterpreted as nagging when it really is not. It is a problem. I think also support from other friends helps.

Q: What about candy bars before vigorous exercise?

Dr Cantu: All right, we have been trying to promote good dietary habits. It is a reality that if you are going to exercise very vigorously, for instance, run 8 to 10 miles, or cross-country ski for an hour and a half, that you are going to burn up more calories than you can really consume with all the salads and fiber and so on you want to eat. There is no harm in a candy bar or two preferably taken before vigorous exercise so that the carbohydrate is burned up during the exercise. Obviously Olympic athletes who are burning 5000 to 6000 calories a day as they train for the Olympics have to fill up with a lot of high-calorie food, and unquestionably for many that means a candy bar or two.

Q: Where can people not in industry get safety glasses for under $10.00?

Dr Vinger: That is a problem in some areas, but most opticians I deal with directly in the Concord-Lexington area do supply safety glasses for slightly above cost, about 12 or 13 dollars.

Q: Are there incidents where it is safe to run through moderate to mild pain such as in a race?

Dr Micheli: Yes, I think that we have all done that. We get concerned when there is real swelling, persistent pain, or atrophy of muscles. Dr Sheehan has often talked about listening to your body so you can tell whether or not you have a serious problem. One of his daughters developed bilateral stress fractures of the tibia. All the time she was listening to her body, so you have to be careful how to listen. I think, though, that you can certainly run with minor pains and irritations without much problem.

Q: Using your data $63.00 per injury and $20.00 for a helmet, would it not be cheaper for insurance companies to voluntarily offer programs, free helmets, or cheaper rates for programs in which they use helmets?

Dr Tolpin: Certainly it would be.

Q: Why do not insurance companies or third party-mechanisms begin to try to offer financial incentives for people to take care of themselves? Why do we not have a system of health insurance payment mechanism (reimbursement mechanism) that would make it expensive for people not to take care of themselves and not to protect themselves when the opportunity is present?

Dr Tolpin: I think the answer is that as long as the insurance company can, by raising their premiums, cover the cost of the liabilities that they incur when people are injured or sick, and as long as the public is willing to pay those insurance premiums, then the insurance companies will continue the status quo.

Q: There are a number of questions here all asking about training programs. Define the need; what kind of a sequence do you actually go through?

Dr Arnot: What I would like to do is indicate what we have been doing in terms of general principles, with our Olympic Cross-country Ski Team, also people just starting out on a fitness program. First, let us discuss volume. We prescribe a certain amount of training. We found that you have to have long-term goals. For the cross-country skier, it is about 2000 km for the first year that they are going to be competing. For an individual jogging for fitness, it might be two to four miles, three times a week. We make absolutely sure they are able to sustain that volume of training without any musculoskeletal symptoms, no aches, no pains, no tendinitis. Then, we start to look at hard-day/easy-day training schedules. It is important to emphasize that, in terms of the cardiovascular training effect, intensity may not be as important as previously thought. Certainly, the longshoremen studies seem to indicate that if you document what changed the heart, it is primarily the basic volume of training.

If you are trying to be reasonably competitive or just want to get a little bit faster, what do you do? Unfortunately, the two things most do are 1) increase the volume of training, and 2) start interval training. They are the wrong things to do. If you are comfortable at 30 or 40 miles a week, that is something you ought to maintain. While maintaining the same distance, start to insert tempo or interval training. While an increase in distance will not make you faster, tempo training will. Each year we might consider an increase in the amount of volume an athlete does of approximately 15% to 20%, whether it is a cross-country skier or runner.

For a competitive program, we emphasize tempo training at a level just below the anaerobic threshold every third day. The tempo is increased each two- to three-week period. It is difficult to know the anaerobic threshold without blood tests that are impractical for most. Fortunately, except for the elite competitive athlete, it is unimportant and the tests should probably be avoided. For the fitness advocate, the talk test is pretty appropriate. Exert at a level where you can still carry on a conversation. For the competitive athletes, you want them to be comfortably winded, just at that point where they are starting to feel out of breath. We give them a sense of that pace by having them run or ski two to three miles to warm up and then start up a long, consistent hill. Each four or five minutes, we increase their pace until they simply cannot maintain it for more than three to four minutes. This is their anaerobic threshold. They are able to get some sense of what the threshold is, this level they do not want to exceed.

I want to repeat that this tempo training is for the competitive athlete. All scientific evidence suggests it is the volume of training that is beneficial in preventing heart attacks. Except for the superbly conditioned, tempo training adds an unacceptable risk of injury.

Q: Dr Childs, why did you not list age and sex as definite risk factors in cardiovascular disease?

Dr Childs: Technically, you are right; they should be on the list. They were not because I admit to a psychological bias. I do not personally see why age and sex need be significant risk factors in cardiovascular disease, and I would like to predict that as time goes by, assuming the things we are talking about become widespread, we will not see them prominently listed.

Q: Do you help your patients select proper aerobic activity and by what criteria?

Dr Childs: If a person comes in, as many do, wanting a specific activity, most often running, the decision is already made and it is simply a matter of is there any reason not to and let's go. If a person really does not seem to be sure, I try hard not to force a person into any given mold, but emphasize the matter of practicality. What a person can do regularly is really the most important factor. You have already seen the list of all the different aerobic activities. A number of them cost quite a bit of money, either in equipment, time, or joining an organization. Those that take a person miles from their home to a place where they have to change and so forth may become a bit of a hassle. So, there are practical hangups that make it hard for people to pick some of the activities, depending upon who they are, where they live, age, economic condition, family situation, and so forth. These are all factors that must be taken into account. I like to have a person make up his or her own mind, what seems most reasonable. Then, once they get started, watch and see what happens. If the person is having trouble, sputtering and fizzling and it just is not working for him, I will begin fairly soon to gently suggest other programs or guide him into a different aerobic activity. I think that practicality has to be the ultimate determinant.

Q: Do you feel a chiropractor has a legitimate claim to a position on the US Olympic Medical Staff?

Dr Cantu: I feel that there is a legitimate place in sports medicine for chiropractice. I realize that every time I say that I darn near get clobbered by 99% of my fellow physicians. I put a qualifier on my contention, that the athlete first be evaluated by an appropriate physician. In other words, I am very disinclined to ever see anybody start with a chiropractor. Chiropractors are not trained in medicine and are not able to diagnose the majority of medical problems and consequently if one starts with a chiropractor, a tumor, ruptured disc, etc may be missed. However, for the individual who has had that particular type of potentially disabling or life-threatening situation eliminated and is left with discomfort, I think that there is a place for a chiropractor preferably working under the direction of, or at least with the supervision of, a physician. Unfortunately, the situation today is that the medical profession treats them with such disdain that the patients seek them out and the doctor never really knows when they are going and what is done. That is a loaded question and this is only a personal opinion; the panel may take issue with it and feel free to comment.

Dr Hoerner: Speaking for myself, I do feel they can be helpful in the treatment of certain mechanical problems. I have two chiropractors working with me.

Dr Micheli: I would basically agree. I know one university sports medicine service that has a chiropractor on the staff. He works very much as Dr Cantu has suggested, under the direction of a physician.

Q: You mentioned an injured eye— should you also patch the uninjured eye to prevent collateral movement?

Dr Vinger: It depends. What we want to do when we patch the eye primarily is to give relief of pain by stopping the lid from blinking and also to stop the patient from doing a forced squeeze. When you normally blink, your eye stays at normal pressure, about 15 mm Hg. When you squeeze your eyes tightly shut, pressure increases to about 17 mm Hg and you could express the contents of a lacerated eye. If you patch both eyes, all you do is panic the injured patient so he tends to thrash about, squeeze, and cause more injury. I know all the first aid books say to patch both eyes, but in practice it usually works better to patch just one.

Q: What are the panel's feelings on the athletic trainers and their role in prevention of injury?

Dr Cantu: I respect their role highly, and believe it is of the utmost importance in the prevention of injuries to athletes. As Dr Vinger said the ultimate responsibility for the prevention of injuries does lie in part with the athlete himself but certainly part of that responsibility has to be shared by the physicians, coaches, and trainers.

Dr Vinger: I think trainers are indispensable, both for the proper administration of the exercises, and for fitting of protective equipment. Many problems arise when protective equipment is fitted improperly. I feel that a major role of trainers should be to ensure this is avoided. As a closing remark, I do not want anybody to think that I am down on sports. I think that they are great; but I would like them to be kept in perspective and have them be as much fun with as little injury as possible.

Dr Micheli: I believe trainers have done a good job of trying to upgrade their training. I think that certification of trainers is something that we must have, and I would hope a certified trainer would be a member of every high school athletic staff.

11 Conclusions

Robert C. Cantu, MD

In this book, we have attempted to present the most current and comprehensive information on a wide range of topics vital to the coach, trainer, physical therapist, nurse, physician, and school and recreational athlete. As the interest and enthusiasm for attaining fitness with its attendant physical and emotional benefits mushroom in popularity, the acute need exists to dispel the many myths, half-truths, and out-and-out quackery. Our faculty, all educators in the health care field, have presented a wealth of concise, factual information with this foremost in mind. Dr Robert Burns Arnot, the exercise physiologist to our Lake Placid Olympic Ski Team, enabled you to understand the physiologic changes that occur with years of endurance training. Describing the changes in the heart, vascular system, and body biochemistry including mitochondrial enhancement and increased anaerobic threshold, increased oxygen transport, and utilization, Dr Arnot showed you how the world-class athlete is built. He also translated all of this for the student or recreational athlete like you or me, and the individual who simply wishes to quietly improve his or her fitness devoid of any group activity or fanfare. In his chapter on corporate fitness, Bob boldly pointed out the challenge to industry to physically shape up, citing both impressive rewards and some risks.

Dr Henry D. Childs, an internist-family physician who specializes in life-style modification, shared his first-hand experience in the frontiers of preventive medicine. Henry brought you into his office for a very down-to-earth look at the ubiquitous ways we may be abusing the most magnificent machines ever constructed, our bodies .And if that does not shock you into change, he points out how some activities, cigarette smoking for instance, are harmful not only to ourselves but to those around us, constituting a form of "child abuse." With the goal of improving the quality of life through aerobic exercise, proper diet, and restraint in self-pollutants, Dr Childs gave an extremely sensitive but forceful message.

For those into jogging and competitive athletics, the chapter by Dr Lyle J. Micheli on the prevention of running and other musculotendinous injuries is a must. Dr Micheli, the Director of Harvard's Sports Medicine Service at Children's Hospital in Boston, helped us to understand what we are doing to our musculoskeletal system, how we place it at risk, and what we can do to avoid injury. With his extremely lucid manner and numerous illustrations, Dr Micheli covered an area vital to any exercise program.

Dr Harriet G. Tolpin, an economist at Simmons College in Boston, afforded insight into the staggering health care costs that injuries and poor life-style create. Dr Tolpin showed how to compute the savings obtained with protective equipment. She also touched on why the insurance companies, as long as premiums can be ever increased, will never be a driving force in the fitness movement.

Dr Paul Vinger, Massachusetts' Ophthalmologist of the Year in 1979, described and illustrated the protective face and eye equipment whose invention he stimulated. Dr Vinger is directly responsible for the mandatory hockey helmets with face masks now worn by all children in amateur organized hockey. Because of his crusade for face and eye protection in sports, not only are millions of health care dollars saved annually, but more importantly countless suffering and even loss of sight are averted.

From his vast clinical experience as Chief of the Sports Medicine Service at Braintree Hospital, Braintree, Massachusetts, Dr Earl Hoerner gave a comprehensive review of upper extremity injuries, their prevention, and treatment. The bio-chemical causes of shoulder, elbow, wrist, and hand injuries were lucidly presented from the common "Little League elbow" and Colles wrist fracture to the less prevalent "snapping shoulder syndrome." Dr Hoerner also described the means of correctly diagnosing these injuries and included many photographs of the actual pathology. Dr Hoerner cautions that pre-adolescent and adolescent athletes are not miniature adults, as they are physically immature. For all athletes, he advocates a year-round training program consisting of three parts: first, cardiovascular and pulmonary fitness; second, flexibility and agility exercises; third, a weight-training program for strength, power, and speed.

In no area is there more hype and quackery than nutrition, a multibillion dollar industry. While the unknown far exceeds the known, in Chapter 4 I gave you what hard facts are known as regards the special nutritional needs of the vigorously exercising. I have an open mind to the omnipresent claims made regarding virtually every known foodstuff, mineral, or vitamin; however, I let you know where scientific verification ends and unproven theories begin.

In the chapter on head and spine injuries prevention , I gave you the knowledge of what are the most hazardous pursuits as well as detailed illustrated exercise programs to alleviate the risk of injury, and for rehabilitation from injury. As is true for most of the leading causes of death and disability, most head and spine injuries are preventable. Though shared by coaches, trainers, and team physicians, the ultimate responsibility for preventing head and spine injuries lies with the athlete himself or herself.

So true, to requote Machiavelli, "fortune is the arbiter of half the things we do, leaving the other half or so to be controlled by ourselves." Today is the first day of the rest of your life and for a happier, more productive, and illness-free future, I beseech you to practice what you have just read.

PROTECTIVE EQUIPMENT SUPPLIERS

Manufacturers of Hockey Face Shields

Fine-mesh, full-face wire shield is recommended as the most durable, probably safest, design style available at this time. Form-fitting goalie face masks are not recommended. Goalies should wear a helmet/full-face wire cage combination for best total head protection. Face shields should be certified either by the Hockey Equipment Certification Council (HECC) or the Canadian Standards Association (CSA).

CCM
2015 Lawrence Avenue West
Weston, Ontario M9N 1H6 Canada

Cooper
501 Alliance Avenue
Toronto, Ontario M6N 2J3
Canada

Jofa, Volvo of American Corp.
Recreational Products Division
266 Union Street
Northvale, NJ 07647

Northland Group, Inc.
124 Columbia Court
Chaska, MN 55318

Pro-Tec, Inc.
11108 Northrup Way
Bellevue, WA 98004

Safe-T-Guard
P.O. Box 934
Madison, WI 53701

St. Lawrence Steel & Wire
81 Mill Street
Gananoque, Ontario K7G 2L5
Canada

Sherbrooke
60 Ellsworth Street
Worcester, MA 01813

Winn Well Limited
113 Sterling Road
Toronto, Ontario M6R 2G9
Canada

Manufacturers of Protective Eyewear for Racquet and Other Sports

Ektelon
8929 Aero Drive
San Diego, CA 92123

Pro-Tec
11108 Northrup Way
Bellevue, WA 98004

Bausch and Lomb
Rochester, NY 14602

Manufacturers of Athletic Frames

American Optical Corp.
Southbridge, MA 01550

Bausch and Lomb
Rochester, NY 14602

Criss Optical Mfg. Co., Inc.
Augusta, KS 67010

Cunningham Sales Corp.
1661 Worcester Road
Framingham, MA 01701

Safety Plastics of New York
(Odyssey Optics)
P.O. Box 47
Eastmeadow, NY 11554

Custom Swim and Diving Goggles, Specialty Optical Work

SEE LAB
William J. Wilber, Jr.
69 Pleasant Street
Manchester-by-the-Sea, MA 01944

Notes:
1. *Protective devices decrease but do not eliminate the chance of injury.*
2. *The above recommendations are subject to change pending future data.*
3. *Some manufacturers of good protective devices may have been inadvertently omitted.*

INDEX

Framingham Study, 57

Glycogen, 10, 12, 45
Golf ball, blow from, 92
Gymnasts, 2, 115, 136, 157

Handball, 157
Hang glider, 157
Harvard Track Team, 13
Health care costs, 74-85
Heart, 2-7
Heart attack, 41, 47, 48
Helmets, 92, 124, 129, 130, 132
Herbert, Victor, 50
High-fiber diet, 58-60
High-pressure work loads, 40
Hips, 70
Hockey masks, 85-86
Homocysteine theory, 53-56
Human Population Library,
  California Health Department,
  37
Hyperlipidemia, 18, 23
Hypertension, 26

Ice hockey, 81-82, 83, 92, 99-
  100
Ignatovski, I.A., 57
Illness, 50-51
Insurance, 39, 78, 166
Institute for Work Physiology
  (Stockholm, Sweden), 3
Intestines, 51

Jogging, 31, 37, 39

Kidney stones, 53
Krebs cycle, 9, 11, 12

Lacrosse, 92
Lactation, 50-51, 54
Lactic acid, 10-12, 40
"Last Chance Diet," 45-46

Lesions, 121, 137
Life-style analysis, 20-22
Lind, James, 52
Lipoprotein, 23, 47, 58
"Little League elbow," 115, 117-
  118
Liver, 48, 50
Lou Harris Poll, 36-37

McCully, Kilmer, 53
McGovern Committee, 44
Mann, George, 56
Maximum oxygen consumption,
  5-7, 13-14
Mayo Clinic, 57
Medical World News, 27
Mitochondria, 9-10
Muscle injury, 65-67, 68, 107-
  122
"Muscle pull," 66
Muscular fatigue, 36
Myocardial infarction, 26
Myositis ossifans, 107

National Center for Health
  Statistics, 132
National Electronic Injuries Sur-
  veillance System (NEISS), 90
National Institutes of Health, 57
National Operating Committee
  on Standards for Athletic Equip-
  ment (NOCSAE), 129
National Society for the Preven-
  tion of Blindness, 90
Neck injuries, 125
New England Journal of
  Medicine, 46, 56
New England Running, 39

Occidental Life of North
  Carolina, 39
Olympics, 1, 132, 135
Osgood-Schlatter disease, 68, 115